Probiotic Ice Cream

Science and Technology

Aziz Homayouni-Rad
Tabriz University of Medical Sciences
Tabriz
Iran

WILEY

This edition first published 2025

Registered Office(s)
John Wiley & Sons, Inc., 111 River Street, Hoboken, NJ 07030, USA
John Wiley & Sons Ltd, The Atrium, Southern Gate, Chichester, West Sussex, PO19 8SQ, UK

For details of our global editorial offices, customer services, and more information about Wiley products visit us at www.wiley.com.

Wiley also publishes its books in a variety of electronic formats and by print-on-demand. Some content that appears in standard print versions of this book may not be available in other formats.

Library of Congress Cataloging-in-Publication Data Applied for

Hardback: 9781119081166

Cover Design: Wiley
Cover Image: © Tetiana Tychynska/Shutterstock, © ADDICTIVESTOCK/Adobe Stock Photos, © Barbara Neveu/Shutterstock, © Rimma Bondarenko/Shutterstock, © Marxstudio/Shutterstock, © Teri Virbickis/Shutterstock, © Roger Bruce/Shutterstock, © Marko Beric/Alamy Stock Photo, © Wavebreak Media ltd/AlamyStock Photo

Set in 9.5/12.5pt STIXTwoText by Straive, Chennai, India

*To my wife (*Mina*) and my daughter (*Sarina*)*

Contents

Preface

Ice cream, a delicious dairy food, is known for its high nutritional value and has been enjoyed as a frozen dessert for many years. Today, the ice cream industry has undergone significant development, and the technology of ice cream production, preservation, and distribution has become an advanced indicator of a country's progress. Various types of ice creams are produced worldwide, including low-fat ice cream, full-fat ice cream, regular ice cream, lactose-free ice cream, probiotic ice cream (Functional), powdered ice cream, sorbet, and fruit-flavored ice creams, each available in different flavors, colors, and shapes. Low-fat ice cream has become common, especially in advanced societies where calorie reduction in their diet is of utmost importance, and its consumption continues to rise. On the other hand, due to lactose intolerance, which results from a lack of the lactase enzyme in the digestive system, people in many parts of the world avoid consuming dairy products containing lactose. In such cases, lactose-free ice cream can be used without causing any problem. Additionally, probiotic ice cream has medicinal properties. The microorganisms present in this type of ice cream can eliminate harmful microbes in the digestive system, and improve consumer health. As a result, the production of this type of product is crucial, particularly in developing countries. Probiotic science and technology has been an ever-growing field in recent decades. Thus, it has opened new vistas of potential research in fermented food formulation and manufacturing. This book is compiled into three sections with 14 chapters highlighting different aspects varying from selection of appropriate probiotic strains for use in ice cream to formulation and characterization of final product. It is designed fundamentally to be a reference book to the experts providing a passage for future researches. So, this book may fill up the gap between probiotic science and probiotic technology in order to manufacturing probiotic ice cream and frozen dairy products. The current book has been written to enhance the knowledge of food industry students and all technical authorities, production managers, ice cream factory owners, operators, technicians, and even employees engaged in these factories. It encompasses generalities, ice cream composition and sources of its constituent parts, ice cream production stages, chemical, physical, and rheological properties of ice cream mix, sensory evaluation of ice cream, methods of producing probiotic ice cream, and quality control of the final product. The coherence of the text owes much to revisions, efforts, and contributions from individuals such as Mrs. Mina Javadi and Mrs. Kosar Tagavi. Also, Mr. Mohammadreza Ziavand and Mrs Sanaz Kazemi worked on figures and tables. Gratitude and appreciation are extended to all these esteemed individuals for their valuable inputs.

Dr. Aziz Homayouni-Rad

Biography

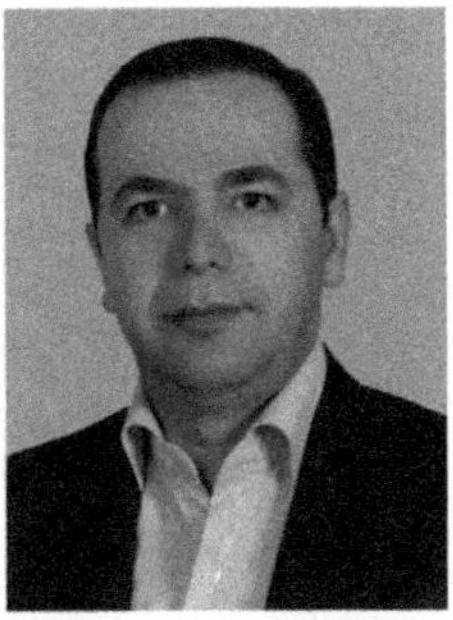

Dr. Aziz Homayouni-Rad obtained his doctoral degree in Food Science and Technology Engineering from Tehran University between 2003 and 2007. Presently, he serves as a professor at Tabriz University of Medical Sciences. He has effectively fulfilled administrative duties as the Vice Chancellor of Education within the Faculty of Nutrition. His research interest is functional foods, with a particular focus on probiotic, prebiotic, synbiotic, and postbiotic dairy products. His notable contributions in this field have earned him numerous accolades and distinctions, including the "Top Researcher in the Faculty of Nutrition at Tabriz University of Medical Sciences in 2013," the "Journal of Dairy Science Most-Cited Award in Dairy Foods in 2014," and "Top 1% most cited researchers of the Essential Science Indicators (ESI) ranking system." His scholarly output comprises over 160 research papers and more than 12 authored books. Additionally, he holds membership in the Iranian Probiotic Association.

Part I

The Science of Probiotic Ice Cream

1

Ice Cream and Frozen Dairy Desserts: Classification and History

1.1 History of Ice Cream Making

In the 13th century, Marco Polo brought formulations of several types of ice cream from Asia to Europe. Therefore, the history of ice cream dates back much further in Asia than in other parts of the world. The art of ice cream making was introduced to Italy by Marco Polo, and from there, it spread to France, Germany, and England, eventually reaching the Americans. The first ice cream-making machine was invented by Marshall in the 19th century (Figure 1.1). In the year 1851 AD, the first ice cream factory was established in the United States by Jacob Fussell, and this marked the transition of ice cream making from an artisanal practice to an industrial one, leading to rapid growth and development. However, around the 1920s, the nutritional value of ice cream gained widespread recognition, and after World War II, the ice cream industry experienced significant expansion.

In the early 20th century, ice cream production expanded and became industrialized due to key factors such as advancements in production techniques, transportation of ice cream, and the preservation of the cold chain. The proliferation of refrigeration machines led to the replacement of salt and ice with a concentrated salt solution (which freezes easily at subzero temperatures). This solution increased the heat transfer rate between the ice cream mixture and the refrigeration unit, thereby boosting production speed. In continuous freezers, which take the form of a horizontal cylinder, the mixture was pumped in from one side and the ice cream was dispensed from the other side, resulting in a more consistent and rapid production compared to discontinuous systems. Such advancements were accompanied by the introduction of pasteurization (which mitigated hygiene concerns) and homogenization (which broke down fat into small droplets, resulting in creamier and smoother products). Eventually, the expansion of railway and

Probiotic Ice Cream: Science and Technology, First Edition. Aziz Homayouni-Rad.

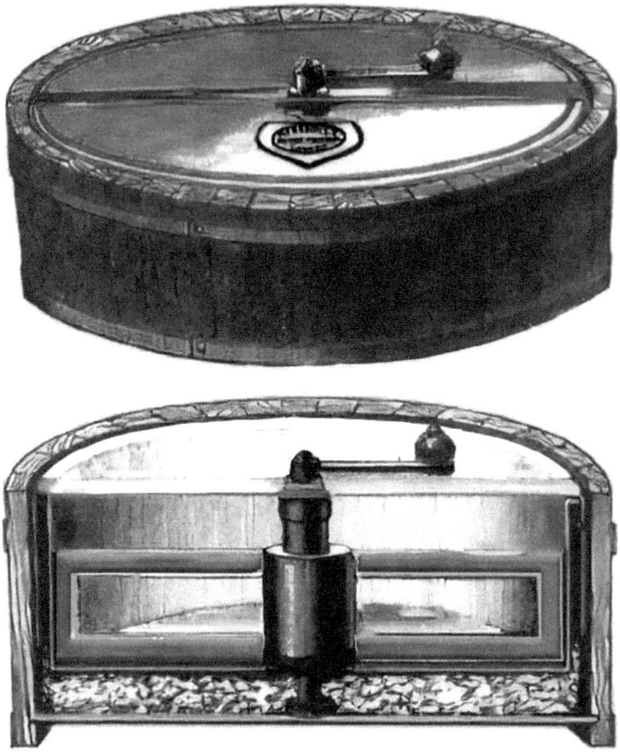

Figure 1.1 The first ice cream-making machine was invented by Marshall in the 19th century.

automobile networks facilitated better transportation of raw materials and distribution of products over longer distances. In Iran, the first ice cream shop located next to a railway track dates back to the reign of Mozaffar al-Din Shah.

1.2 Definition of Ice Cream

Ice cream is a frozen food product made from cow's milk and can contain permissible edible ingredients such as sugar, dextrose, eggs, fruits, fruit juices, chocolate, nuts, flavorings, and food-grade colorings. Emulsifiers and stabilizers can also be used in its composition. The composition of ice cream varies from one region to another. Generally, a good ice cream contains around 12% fat, 11% nonfat milk solids, 15% sugar, 0.3% stabilizers

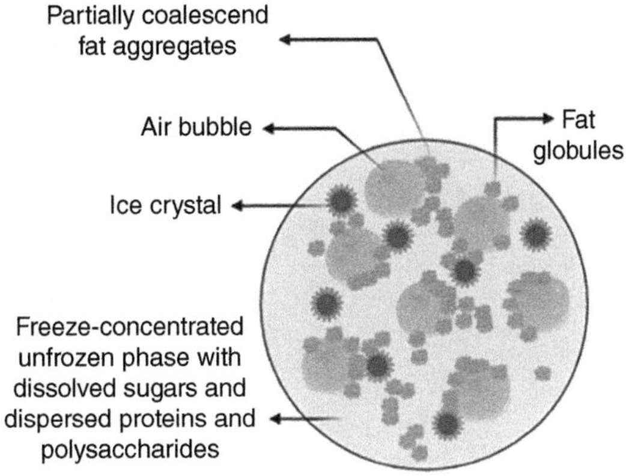

Figure 1.2 Schematic structure of ice cream; ice crystals, air bubbles, fat globules, and serum phase.

and emulsifier mixture, and a total of 38% dry matter. Ice cream is a complex composition of three phases: the gas, solid, and liquid phases. The gas phase consists of air bubbles uniformly distributed in the frozen phase. The liquid phase contains frozen fat globules, milk proteins, insoluble salts, colloidal stabilizers, sugars, and soluble salts. Thus, the final product is a three-phase system consisting of liquid, solid, and gas (Figure 1.2).

Ice cream is a highly delicious and nutritious food. Approximately, 100 grams of good-quality ice cream provides around 200 kilocalories of energy, along with 4 grams of protein, 0.13 grams of calcium, 0.105 grams of phosphorus, 0.1 gram of iron, 490 IU of vitamin A, 0.38 milligrams of thiamine, and 0.24 milligrams of riboflavin. The production and consumption levels of ice cream in some countries around the world are presented in Table 1.1.

1.3 Classification of Ice Cream

Various factors such as raw materials, consumer preferences, costs, and quality influence the formulation of different ice cream mixes. The percentage of stabilizers and emulsifiers required in different mixtures varies, and therefore the usage of these components should adhere to the manufacturer's recommendations. Ice cream can be classified based on brand name, ingredients, and flavoring agents used. Below, different types of ice cream and similar products are categorized using commercial methods. The formulation of regular ice cream is provided in Table 1.2.

Please note that the percentages provided here represent a hypothetical formulation for regular ice cream and are subject to variations based on specific recipes and manufacturing processes.

Table 1.1 Major ice cream-producing and consuming countries in the world.

Top ice cream-producing countries:

Rank	Production (Million hectoliters per year)	Country
1	26.3	New Zealand
2	8.17	Australia
3	8.17	Canada
4	8.1	Italy
5	4.14	Sweden
6	2.14	Denmark
7	9.13	Finland
8	2.9	Switzerland
9	2.8	China
10	4.5	France
11	8.3	Germany
12	2.3	United States

Top ice cream-consuming countries:

Rank	Consumption (Liters per capita per year)	Country
1	26.3	New Zealand
2	22.5	United States
3	17.8	Canada
4	17.6	Australia
5	14.4	Switzerland
6	14.2	Sweden
7	13.9	Finland
8	9.2	Denmark
9	8.2	Italy
10	5.4	France
11	3.8	Germany
12	1.8	China

Data represents a specific time period and may have changed since then.

Table 1.2 Formulation of regular ice creams.

Percentage of ingredients	Regular ice cream formulation (1)
Fat	18
Nonfat milk solids	7
Sugar	18
Stabilizers	0.2
Total solids	43.2

Percentage of ingredients	Regular ice cream formulation (2)
Fat	16
Nonfat milk solids	8.5
Sugar	17
Stabilizers	0.25
Total solids	41.75

Percentage of ingredients	Regular ice cream formulation (3)
Fat	14
Nonfat milk solids	10
Sugar	15
Stabilizers	0.3
Total solids	39.3

Percentage of ingredients	Regular ice cream formulation (4)
Fat	12
Nonfat milk solids	11
Sugar	15
Stabilizers	0.3
Total solids	38.3

Percentage of ingredients	Regular ice cream formulation (5)
Fat	10
Nonfat milk solids	11.5
Sugar	15
Stabilizers	0.3
Total solids	36.8

1.3.1 Regular Ice Cream Types

Regular ice cream is a type of ice cream in which the total volume of flavoring and coloring ingredients is less than 5%. Examples of this type include vanilla ice cream, coffee ice cream, caramel ice cream, and orange ice cream. The following section provides explanations of various types of regular ice cream:

Coffee Ice Cream:
To make coffee ice cream, you add 0.946 liters of coffee extract (or you can use a concentrated coffee extract obtained from 453.6 grams of ground coffee) to 37.85 liters of the regular ice cream mixture. Additionally, you can add 141.75–198.45 grams of color derived from 50% burnt sugar (caramel) to enhance the flavor.

Vanilla Ice Cream:
For producing vanilla ice cream, you include 170.1–340.2 grams of flavoring ingredients and 8 milliliters of yellow color to every 37.85 liters of the regular ice cream mixture. The actual amount of flavoring may vary based on the mixture's composition, individuals' preferences, and the desired intensity of the vanilla flavor.

Saffron Ice Cream:
To prepare saffron ice cream, you add 85.05 grams of pure saffron extract and 56.7 grams of caramel to every 37.85 liters of the regular ice cream mixture.

Caramel Ice Cream:
You add an appropriate amount of caramel to achieve the desired taste and color for caramel ice cream. Alternatively, you can use 2.838 liters of caramel syrup for every 35 liters of the regular ice cream mixture (approximately 113.4 grams of syrup per 3.785 liters of ice cream). To make caramel syrup, a mixture of 5 parts sugar and 3 parts 20% fat cream is boiled until a light coffee color is achieved.

Mint Ice Cream:
To create mint ice cream, you incorporate 113.4–226.8 grams of mint extract and add green color to achieve a light green hue to every 37.85 liters of the regular ice cream mixture. Sometimes, 1814.4–2721.6 grams of chopped green mint mixture can be added to 35/95 liters of the regular ice cream mixture.

Butterscotch Ice Cream:
In this type of ice cream, you add 3.785 liters of butterscotch syrup, which is used in the production of butterscotch pastries, to 37.85 liters of the regular ice cream mixture. Additionally, a yellow color is added along with the syrup.

Bisque Ice Cream:

For making bisque ice cream, you combine 1814.4–3628.8 grams of starch noodles, sponge cake, finger sweets, grapes, cookie dough, brownie, or similar small and finely chopped ingredients with 35.95 liters of the regular ice cream mixture. These additions are made through a noncontinuous freezer.

Creamy Sweet Ice Cream (Biscuit, Tortoni):

In this type of ice cream, you blend 0.473 liters of dark brown sugar syrup or ingredients that contribute to the flavor with 37.85 liters of high-fat (14–17% fat) ice cream mixture. The mixture can be expanded by a maximum of 50% (overrun) of its frozen volume, and after filling, crushed starch noodles are added on top.

Candy or Confection Ice Cream:

There are many types of ice creams with various names and flavors in this category. These types of ice creams contain 5–8% of different types of confections or candies. These confections and nonsoluble additives are usually added to the unfrozen ice cream using noncontinuous freezers. Additionally, it is possible to continuously add raw materials to a product that is in the process of freezing using a feeding device. The various types of these ice creams are as follows:

(A) **Butter Paste Ice Cream:** 2721.6 grams of crumbled butter bread are added to 35.95 liters of regular ice cream mixture.

(B) **Chocolate Ice Cream:** 1.892 liters of grated milk chocolate or milk chocolate syrup are added to 35.95 liters of regular ice cream mixture. The chocolate is added to the ice cream that has partially frozen in a noncontinuous freezer.

(C) **Peanut Ice Cream:** 1814.4–2721.6 grams of chopped peanut particles are added to 35.95 liters of regular ice cream mixture.

(D) **Marshmallow Ice Cream:** 1814.4–2721.6 grams of marshmallow (a sweet dough containing sugar, starch, and corn syrup) are added to 35.95 liters of regular ice cream mixture.

(E) **Chocolate Powder Ice Cream:** 1814.4–2721.6 grams of milk chocolate powder are added to 35.95 liters of regular ice cream mixture.

(F) **Licorice Ice Cream:** 113.4 grams of licorice paste and 36.85 grams of fennel oil are added to 35.95 liters of regular ice cream mixture until a dark color is achieved.

(G) **Molasses Ice Cream:** 1814.4–2721.6 grams of molasses are added to 35.95 liters of regular ice cream mixture.

(H) **Toffee Ice Cream:** 1814.4–2721.6 grams of chopped toffee is added to 35.95 liters of regular ice cream mixture. To prepare the toffee, a mixture of 907.2 grams of butter and 2268 grams of sugar is heated to

160°C, and after removing from heat, half a tablespoon of baking soda is added. The mixture is thoroughly mixed, then mixed with 680.4 grams of nuts, spread, and dried.

(I) **Ginger Ice Cream:** 3628.8 grams of chopped ginger root jam is added to 35.95 liters of regular ice cream.

1.3.2 Chocolate Ice Cream

Chocolate ice cream is flavored with cocoa or chocolate. The required amounts of cocoa to create the chocolate flavor using a mixture of cocoa and chocolate syrup, chocolate syrup, and chocolate are 1587.6–2041.2, 2494.8, 1224.72–1360.8 grams per 37.85 liters of ice cream mixture, respectively. Different types of chocolate ice cream are described below. The chocolate ice cream formulation is presented in Table 1.3.

Simple Chocolate Ice Cream: Chocolate syrup is added to 34 liters of regular ice cream mixture. This chocolate syrup is prepared from 1360.8 grams of cocoa or 1814.4 grams of chocolate syrup, 1360.8 grams of sugar, and 3/78–5/67 liters of water. Sugar and cocoa are mixed together, and enough water is added to them to form a paste. Then, it is heated with steam in a double-walled vessel. As the syrup thickens, water is gradually added while continuously stirring. It is then heated up to a temperature of 80°C and after being discharged, it is cooled down for use. The required amount of water prevents the syrup from thickening excessively.

Mint Chocolate Ice Cream: 1814.4–2721.6 grams of dried mint leaves are added to 35.95 liters of regular ice cream mixture.

Malt Chocolate Ice Cream: To 34 liters of regular ice cream mixture, half of the chocolate syrup is used for chocolate ice cream and 0.946 liter of malt syrup is added. If malt syrup is not available, 453.6–907.2 grams of malted milk can be used instead.

Table 1.3 Chocolate ice cream formulation.

Ingredient percentage	Chocolate ice cream				
Fat	16	14	12	10	8
Nonfat milk solids	8	10	11	12	12.5
Sugar	19	17	16	16	16
Cocoa	3.5	3	3	3	2.7
Stabilizers	0.2	0.25	0.25	0.3	0.3
Total solids	46.7	44.25	42.25	41.3	39.5

Chocolate Almond Ice Cream: 1814.4–2721.6 grams of chopped almond is added to 35.95 liters of chocolate ice cream mixture.

Chocolate Marshmallow Ice Cream: 1814.4–2721.6 grams of marshmallow is added to 35.95 liters of chocolate ice cream mixture.

Chocolate Coffee Ice Cream: To 28.38 liters of regular ice cream mixture, 9.46 liters of chocolate mixture and 226.8–340.2 grams of coffee syrup or sufficient coffee extract are added to create a mild coffee flavor in the product.

1.3.3 Fruit Ice Cream

Fruit ice cream contains actual fruit and can also include fruit essence and coloring. Fruits like pineapple, apricot, strawberry, etc., whether fresh, frozen, or in conserved form, can be used in fruit ice cream. Fruit ice creams can be flavored by incorporating 10–15% fruit into regular ice cream mixtures, where the type of fruit and desired intensity of flavor influence the amount of fruit used. When using frozen fruit for making fruit ice cream, the fruit-to-sugar ratio varies between 1:2.5 and 1:4. The type of fruit also plays a determining role in formulation. Various types of fruit ice creams are described below:

Strawberry Ice Cream: To 30.28 liters of regular ice cream mixture, 7.57 liters of processed aseptic strawberry puree is added. In this type of ice cream, fruit is used in the form of puree and is firm, and to achieve a desirable yellow color, a certain amount of red color is also added.

Peach Ice Cream: To 30.28 liters of regular ice cream mixture, 7.57 liters of fruit is added. To enhance the intensity of flavor and color, a portion of this fruit should be in the form of puree. The color of the ice cream should be light yellow.

Cherry Ice Cream: To 32.17–34 liters of regular ice cream mixture, 3.78–5.67 liters of cherry is added. Sour cherry concentrate should be used to improve the taste. The color of this ice cream should be light red.

Apricot Ice Cream: To 30.28 liters of regular ice cream mixture, 7.57 liters of apricot is added. The color of this ice cream should be light yellow.

Apple Ice Cream: To 30.28 liters of regular ice cream mixture, 7.57 liters of chopped apples are added. Frozen apples should be packed with a 1:7 ratio of sugar. The apple flavor can be enhanced by adding 320 milliliters of apple essence to the ice cream.

Pineapple Ice Cream: To 34 liters of regular ice cream mixture, 3.785 liters of grated pineapple are added.

Banana Ice Cream: To 34 liters of regular ice cream mixture, 3.785 liters of grated banana are added. If fresh bananas are used, they should be fully ripe. Adding a small amount of citric acid or lemon juice can prevent browning of fresh fruit and improve its taste.

Orange Ice Cream: To 34 liters of regular ice cream mixture, 3.785 liters of orange juice and 0.946 liters of lemon juice are added. Additionally, 1360.8 grams of fruit sugar is added at the beginning. The color of this ice cream should be light orange.

Orange and Pineapple Mixed Ice Cream: To 34 liters of regular ice cream mixture, 3.785 liters of grated pineapple and sufficient concentrated orange juice are added to create an orange flavor. The color of this ice cream should be light orange.

Lemon Ice Cream: To 34 liters of regular ice cream mixture, 3.785 liters of fresh or frozen lemon juice, 0.946 liters of orange juice, and 1360.8 grams of sugar are added. The color of this ice cream should be lemon yellow.

Mulberry Ice Cream: To 34 liters of regular ice cream mixture, 3.785 liters of black or red mulberry puree with sugar (in equal proportions) are added. Adding mulberry extract is essential to enhance the flavor.

Fig and Nut Ice Cream: To 34 liters of regular ice cream mixture, 3.785 liters of canned figs and 907.2 grams of chopped nuts are added. The color of this ice cream should be light brown.

Grape Ice Cream: To 34 liters of regular ice cream mixture, 3.785 liters of concentrated grape juice are added.

Blueberry Ice Cream: To 30.28 liters of regular ice cream mixture, 7.57 liters of blueberry puree are added.

Vanilla Cherry Ice Cream: To 30.28 liters of regular ice cream mixture, 7.57 liters of intact cherries (without damage and stems removed) are added. Fruits are added using a special feeder for raw materials.

Date Ice Cream: To 30.28 liters of regular ice cream mixture, 7.57 liters of chopped dates are added.

1.3.4 Nutty Ice Cream

This type of ice cream contains nuts such as almonds, walnuts, pistachios, etc., and can also include flavorings for both color and taste enhancement. A regular ice cream mixture with 10–14% fat content can be made flavorful by adding 3–6% nuts. Buttery and caramel flavors are commonly used. Various types of nutty ice cream are described below:

Nutty Ice Cream with Toasted Almond Flavor: To 35.95 liters of regular ice cream mixture, 1814.4–2268 grams of toasted or roasted almonds are added. Almond flavoring and caramel colorings are also used.

Pistachio-Flavored Nutty Ice Cream: To 35.95 liters of regular ice cream mixture, 1814.4 grams of chopped pistachios and pistachio extract (enough to create a flavor and light green color) are added.

Creamy Walnut-Flavored Nutty Ice Cream: To 35.95 liters of regular ice cream mixture, 1360.8 grams of special buttery sweet (that creates a crunchy sound when chewed) and 907.2 grams of chopped walnuts are added. This type of ice cream can also be prepared using 34 liters of the regular mixture and 4536 grams of walnut, either coarsely ground, finely milled, or a mix of the two.

Walnut-Flavored Nutty Ice Cream with Maple Syrup: To 35.95 liters of regular ice cream mixture, 907.2–1360.8 grams of chopped walnuts and 85 grams of pure maple extract are added.

Walnut-Flavored Nutty Ice Cream: To 35.95 liters of regular ice cream mixture, 1814.4–2268 grams of chopped walnuts are added.

Caramel-Flavored Nutty Ice Cream: To 35.95 liters of regular ice cream mixture, 1360.8 grams of chopped nuts, 56.7 grams of caramelized sugar (for color), and caramel flavorings are added.

Nutty Pineapple Ice Cream: To 34 liters of regular ice cream mixture, 3.785 liters of pineapple and 1360.8 grams of chopped nuts are added.

Walnut Crunch Ice Cream: To 35.95 liters of regular ice cream mixture, 2721.6 grams of ground candy with chopped walnuts are added.

Banana Nutty Ice Cream: To 35.95 liters of regular ice cream mixture, 2.84 liters of grated bananas and 907.2 grams of chopped nuts are added.

Chocolate Almond Ice Cream: To 35.95 liters of chocolate ice cream mixture, 1814.4 grams of whole or chopped almonds are added.

Toffee Almond Ice Cream: To 35.95 liters of regular ice cream mixture, 1814.4 grams of chopped buttery toffee and 907.2 grams of chopped almonds are added.

Pineapple and Coconut Nutty Ice Cream: To 34 liters of regular ice cream mixture, 2.84 liters of grated pineapple and 1814.4 grams of chopped coconut are added.

Peanut-Flavored Nutty Ice Cream: To 35.95 liters of regular ice cream mixture, 1814.4–2721.6 grams of chopped peanuts or peanut butter are added.

1.3.5 Yoghurt Ice Cream

This type of ice cream mixture is cultured using yoghurt bacteria and may be classified as probiotic ice cream (Homayouni 2008). Fruits, nuts, and various flavoring ingredients can be added to the mixture before or after pasteurization and culturing. Yoghurt ice cream is produced by freezing and simultaneously agitating a pasteurized mixture containing milk fat, nonfat milk solids, sweeteners, and yoghurt. Various flavorings can be used, often incorporating fruits. After pasteurizing the milk, a mixture of *Lactobacillus bulgaricus* and *Streptococcus thermophilus* bacteria is introduced into the yoghurt components. If pasteurization is performed after culturing these bacteria, it needs to be indicated on the product label. Typically, the milk is subjected to high-temperature treatment (e.g., at 85°C for 15 minutes) before inoculating with yoghurt starter. In industrial production, the titratable acidity of the final yoghurt mixture should be 0.30%. Usually, 10–20% yoghurt (by weight) is used in the mixture. To mitigate the tangy flavor of regular yoghurt, efforts are made to reduce the level of acetaldehyde taste in yoghurt ice cream. The tangy taste of yoghurt is slightly more pronounced compared to low-fat ice cream, even when the fat content of both is the same. The increased attention toward yoghurt ice cream compared to other frozen dairy products is due to the belief that yoghurt bacteria aid lactose digestion and offer other immune-modulating properties. Yoghurt ice cream contains relatively low fat content, and its labeling varies based on the fat content, similar to the nomenclature used for other ice cream types. If it contains less than 0.5 gram of fat per 113 grams serving, it is labeled as "fat-free yoghurt ice cream." If it contains 0.5–3 grams of fat, it is labeled as "low-fat yoghurt ice cream," and if it contains more than 3 grams of fat, it is labeled as "full-fat yoghurt ice cream." The formulation of peach and strawberry-flavored yoghurt ice cream is presented in Tables 1.4 and 1.5.

Table 1.4 Formulation of peach-flavored yoghurt ice cream.

Ingredients	Quantity
Regular ice cream mixture (5% fat content)	11.35 liters
Low-fat yoghurt	3.785 liters
Yoghurt stabilizer	3.785 liters
Peach puree	0.473 liters
Peach cubes	1.892 liters
Peach flavor extract	85 grams
Yoghurt acid (lactic acid)	28.35 grams
Citric acid	28.35 grams

Table 1.5 Formulation of strawberry-flavored yoghurt ice cream.

Ingredients	Quantity
Regular ice cream mixture	11.35 liters
Low-fat yoghurt	3.785 liters
Yoghurt stabilizer	3.785 liters
Strawberries	2.13 liters
Frozen strawberries	1.892 liters
Yoghurt acid (lactic acid)	42.525 grams
Citric acid	28.35 grams
Strawberry flavor extract	7.08 grams

1.3.6 Puddings

Nesselrode Pudding: In Nesselrode pudding, 30.28–32.17 liters of regular ice cream mixture with 14–16% fat content are mixed with 5.676–7.568 liters of various commercial fruits. The fruits are added after the mixture has frozen to a certain extent, using a specialized fruit feeder device. The Nesselrode mixture typically includes 0.946 liters of grated pineapple, cherries, cherry preserves, various types of raisins, 340.2 grams of orange peel preserves, and 907.2 grams of chopped almonds and walnuts. The product's color should be light orange, and often, the regular ice cream mixture is used instead of a high-fat mixture for making Nesselrode pudding.

Berry Pudding: To prepare berry pudding, 3.78–7.56 liters of regular ice cream mixture are mixed with a blend of various suitable fruits. The product's color should be light pink. The pudding mixture contains small pieces of red cherries (1.892 liters), shredded pineapple (1.892 liters), and chopped almonds (907.2 grams). It is worth mentioning that red coloring is added to the mixture after it is prepared.

Frozen Pudding: For this type of pudding, nuts, essences, or flavoring ingredients are added to berry ice cream.

Peach Pudding: To 30.28 liters of parfait ice cream mixture (16% fat), after it is slightly frozen, 1360.8 grams of chocolate syrup, various types of fruit and nuts, including 907.2 grams of figs, 907.2 grams of dates, 3628.8 grams of mixed fruit preserves, 907.2 grams of walnuts, 226.8 grams of vanilla extract, 6 tablespoons of cinnamon, and 1 tablespoon of ginger are added. The fruits and nuts should be chopped and mixed with spices before adding to the slightly frozen mixture. Spices are also added before the freezing process begins. Sometimes, for making peach pudding, 30.28 liters of regular ice cream mixture is mixed with 3628.8 grams of egg yolks, 2721.6 grams of sugar, 3.784 liters of orange juice, 1814.4 grams of walnuts, and 226.8 grams of vanilla.

Date Pudding: To 34 liters of regular ice cream mixture, 2721.6 grams of dates and 907.2 grams of chopped walnuts are added.

1.3.7 Special Ice Creams

Egg and Milk Ice Cream: To 34 liters of regular ice cream mixture, 3.785 liters of a mixture of milk and eggs are added. The milk and egg mixture can be prepared using 6804 grams of eggs, 3402 grams of fresh egg yolks, 1814.4 grams of egg powder, 3628.8 grams of sugar, and 204.2 grams of cream (20% fat). This mixture is heated at a temperature of 71°C for 20–30 minutes and then homogenized. This type of ice cream can also be prepared using 37.85 liters of regular ice cream mixture, 680.4 grams of egg yolk powder, 85 grams of vanilla extract, 56.7 grams of lemon juice, 0.45 liters of cane essence, 85 grams of egg yolk color, and various seasonings.

Raisin Fermented Ice Cream: To 34 liters of regular ice cream mixture, 11,340 grams of seedless raisins and 113.4–170.1 grams of fermented syrup or aromatic materials such as cane essence and yellow color are added.

Date and Walnut Ice Cream: To 34 liters of regular ice cream mixture, 6804 grams of dates, 1360.8–1814.4 grams of walnuts, and a certain amount of color are added. Dates and walnuts should be mixed with a little sugar and then added to the ice cream mixture.

Sweet Potato Ice Cream: To 24.5 liters of regular ice cream mixture, 12,700.8 grams of sweet potato puree (1:7 ratio with sugar), 0.946 liters of lemon juice, 56.7 milliliters of vanilla extract, and 113.4 grams of Prussian orange color are added. 1814.4 grams of mashed Avocado is mixed with 453.6 grams of sugar. Then, 7257.6 grams of this mixture is added to 40,824 grams of the previous mixture.

Honey Ice Cream: A well-composed honey ice cream mixture consists of 10% milk fat, 10% nonfat solids, 8% sugar, 9% honey, and 0.3% stabilizers. Using too much honey can lead to freezing and firmness issues. In such cases, using a formulation of 10% milk fat, 1% nonfat solids, 8% low DE (dextrose equivalent) corn syrup, 12% honey, and 0.25% stabilizers can yield a highly flavorful product with sufficient sweetness. Honey with a milder taste and lighter color is preferred in ice cream.

Plum Ice Cream: To 30.28 liters of regular ice cream mixture, 7.57 liters of pureed plum (1:4 ratio with sugar), 0.473 liters of grated orange zest, and 56.7 grams of vanilla are added. Plums should be prepared after peeling and removing the pit from the fruit. Plums give the product a golden yellow color and a soft texture that makes it delicious.

Watermelon Ice Cream: To 37.85 liters of regular ice cream mixture, 283.5–340.2 grams of watermelon-flavoring materials are added. This type of product is pink in color.

Rhubarb Ice Cream: To 32.17 liters of regular ice cream mixture, 5.67 liters of cooked and grated rhubarb (1:3 ratio with sugar), 907.2 grams of chopped walnuts, 0.946 liters of orange slices, 56.7 grams of vanilla, and 14.175 grams of nutmeg flakes are added. This product has a pink color.

Pumpkin Ice Cream: To 30.28 liters of regular ice cream mixture, 7.57 liters of cooked pumpkin puree, 0.946 liters of orange slices, 56.7 grams of vanilla, 14.175 grams of cinnamon, and 7.08 grams of nutmeg flakes are added.

Fruit Cube Ice Cream: For the fruit mixture, dissolve 170.1 grams of flavored gelatin in one cup of water, and mix 567 grams of this product with fruit (typically frozen fruit with sugar). Add 4 eggs, 2 cups of sweetened condensed milk, 1/33 cup of sugar, 1.892 milliliters of corn syrup, and 170.1 grams of vanilla pudding mix. Mix these ingredients together. Then, add the fruit mixture to the ice cream mixture. The resulting mixture, with a volume of 5.676 liters, will be sufficient for freezing in the freezer.

Homemade Ice Cream: By using the ingredients from Table 1.6 along with flavoring materials and freezing the mixture in an ice and salt freezer, one can obtain a gallon of ice cream. Adding a tablespoon of vanilla extract can flavor the mixture. The gelatin used should be dissolved in half a cup of cold water.

Table 1.6 Primary ingredients of homemade ice cream.

Ingredients	Ice cream formulations				
Heavy cream (liter)	1.23	1.23	1.42	1.42	0.946
Milk (liter)	1.42	1.42	1.42	1.42	0.946
Concentrated milk (gr)	385	385	425	425	425
Sugar (glass)	2	2	2	2	2
Gelatin (teaspoon)	1	1	1	1	1

1.3.8 Other Types of Ice Cream

French Custard Ice Cream: This type of ice cream is made using eggs. The weight of solid materials in frozen custard should be less than 1.4, and in unfrozen products, less than 1.2 of the total weight.

Fruit Puree Ice Cream: This type of ice cream includes flavoring ingredients and pieces of fruit candy, such as mint sticks.

Biscuit Ice Cream: This ice cream has a distinct flavor and incorporates ingredients like raisins, sweet breads, cakes, and other bakery products.

Mousse Ice Cream: This ice cream contains whipped cream along with sugar, and coloring and flavoring agents. It receives minimal aeration during freezing and sometimes uses condensed milk to enhance its texture. To make a small quantity of mousse, whip 3.785 milliliters of cream until firm. Then, mix it vigorously with 907.2 grams of sugar, 1–2 drops of suitable color, and 14.175–28.35 grams of vanilla. Small pieces of dates, nuts, and dried fruits are added to the mixture. The mixture is placed in a container and allowed to set without additional whipping. For large-scale production, 22.2 liters of heavy whipped cream, 7.57 liters of milk, 6350.4 grams of sugar, 170.1 grams of stabilizer, and 870.1 grams of vanilla are used. To dissolve the stabilizer, mix it with about 907.2 grams of sugar and blend it with the whipped cream. Heat the milk to the required temperature to dissolve the stabilizer, then combine it with the remaining initial ingredients. Chill the mixture to 0°C, intermittently freezing it to achieve a slight increase in volume before firming it up before consumption.

Rainbow Ice Cream: Vanilla ice cream blended with syrup and chocolate, creating a marbled appearance once hardened.

Gourmet Ice Cream: This type of ice cream usually combines various flavoring ingredients.

Napoleon Ice Cream: Consists of two or more flavors of ice cream packaged together.

Sweetened Ice Cream: A type of ice cream containing 2–7% fat and 12–15% nonfat dry solids, sweeteners, and flavoring agents.

Fruit Ice Cream: Fruit ice cream is made from fruit puree, sugar, stabilizers, and dairy products. It resembles regular ice cream but uses whole milk, reduced-fat milk, condensed milk, dry milk, or a mixture of these instead of all or part of the water content.

Sherbet Ice Cream: This type of ice cream is made from fruit juice, sugar, and stabilizers. It might contain fruit acids, coloring, and flavoring. It attains a suitable texture upon freezing. Typically, 28–30% sugar is used in sherbet formulations. Overrun (the expansion factor) is about 20–25% in sherbets. Dairy products are not used in its formulation.

Soft-Serve Ice Cream: This product is consumed immediately after being dispensed from the freezer, in a soft and creamy state. There is no hardening stage involved.

Novelties Ice Cream: These new types of ice creams are a combination of frozen and semifrozen dairy mixtures, presented in various shapes, sizes, and colors. Examples include Eskimo pies, coated ice cream bars, sandwiched ice creams, and cubed ice cream bars between layers of biscuits that are packaged in waxed paper.

Frappe: A type of chilled product consisting of a blended mixture of fruit-infused water, with a slightly soft and smooth texture. This product is consumed as a cold beverage. Frappé is prepared similar to ice cream, but it is consumed in a soft form. To prepare 18.5 liters of frappé, 4082.4 grams of sugar, 2041.2 grams of solid corn syrup, 85.05 grams of pectin, and 3.785 liters of fruit juice are mixed together, and with enough water (10,409 grams), its volume reaches 18.5 liters. Before consumption, it freezes into a soft mixed texture.

Granite Ice Cream: A type of frozen ice cream that is slightly aerated during freezing. As a result, its overrun is lower. The same ingredients used to prepare regular ice cream are used for making granite. Less aeration and whipping occur during the freezing of granite. This product has a coarser texture compared to regular ice cream.

Souffle Ice Cream: A syrup containing egg yolks or whole eggs.

Lacto: A milk-based syrup that incorporates fermented milk, yoghurt, or cultured milk in its composition. Lacto is prepared from a mixture of fruit-flavored ice cream containing sour milk (cultured), buttermilk, or other cultured dairy products. To produce grape lacto, 11.355 liters of buttermilk, 4082.4 grams of sugar, 680.4 grams of egg yolk, 3 cups of lemon water, and 0.946 liters of grape juice are used. Sugar is dissolved in the milk and grape juice, followed by the addition of egg yolk. The egg white is beaten and added to the mixture, then transferred to a noncontinuous freezer. Instead of grape juice, cranberry, cherry, or orange juice can also be used.

Fruit Salad Ice Cream: A mixture of whipped cream and large fruit pieces that is consumed as a fruit salad after freezing. Mayonnaise sauce can be added when consumed. This product is a combination of large fruit pieces mixed with whipped cream or ice cream. Around 3.785 liters of mixed pineapple, red cherries, apricots, peaches, pears, or plums are combined with 2.52 liters of whipped cream to give it a mayonnaise-like taste. The mixture is left to firm up, and around 2.52 liters of soft ice cream can be used as a substitute for whipped cream. If an 85-gram packet of gelatin is dissolved in a cup of hot water and added to the cold fruit mixture, the volume of the salad increases.

Sculpted Ice Cream: This category includes ice cream, ice, and shaped syrups that are made in single or multiple colors and various flavors, and then decorated. Types of sculpted ice cream include:

(A) Layered cube-shaped ice cream with decorative centers.
(B) Cookie-shaped or cylindrical ice cream.
(C) Cake-shaped tube ice cream.
(D) Ice creams shaped like different fruits, flowers, and animals.
(E) Multilayered ice creams with different colors, where a layer of fruit jam is placed between two ice cream layers or fruit pieces may be added as soon as the ice cream exits the freezer.

Melorin: The formulation of this ice cream is similar to regular ice cream, except that butterfat is replaced with vegetable or animal oils.

Frozen Dairy Products with Artificial Sweeteners: In these products, nonsugar and non-nutritive sweeteners are used instead of sugar.

Nondairy Frozen Desserts: The ingredients of these products are similar to ice cream but without dairy components.

Parfait: For every 7.57 liters of ice cream mix, 16% fat, 1200 grams of egg yolk powder, or 3628.8 grams of whole egg are added. After baking (at 41°C for 30 minutes), it turns into a pastry, which is then cooled to 38°C. This pastry is added to 26.49 liters of the same ice cream mix, and 37.85 liters of the resulting parfait mix is flavored as usual, similar to ice cream.

Frozen Sherbet: It is similar to ice cream but with relatively high sugar content (30%) and consists of 30–50% fruit and fruit juice, pectin, gum stabilizers (0.4%), and usually 2.6% egg white. Its overrun is also 20% or less. Citric acid is added to improve the taste, and water is used to adjust the volume of the mixture.

Punch: Punch is a type of frozen dessert prepared by mixing 26.5 liters of water, 9072 grams of sugar, 0.946 liters of lemon juice, 0.946 liters of grape juice, and some vanilla essence. Adding 141.75 liters of stabilizing agents can freeze the product for consumption.

Soffle: This product is prepared from a mixture of fruit-flavored ice cream to which whole eggs are added. Due to the volume increase during freezing, the product expands. To prepare this product, 28.38 liters of fruit-flavored ice cream mix, 3628.8 grams of whole egg, and 7.57 liters of fruit puree are used.

Fancy Molded Ice Cream: "Ofa" is composed of molded ice cream and fruit, containing two or more layers of ice cream with fruit placed between them. To prepare "Ofa," strawberry is used, which practically encompasses the entire ice cream. It is then allowed to be set and covered with a thin layer of pectin-enriched strawberry. Finally, the mold is filled with vanilla or strawberry ice cream. The fruit should have a viscosity that creates somewhat extended lines in the ice cream, resulting in a marbled appearance of the final product.

Spumoni: Vanilla ice cream is filled into a spumoni cup, about one-fourth of its height, and compressed well against the sides. Then, the cup is filled up to half with chocolate ice cream. In the end, it is topped off with a mixture of fruit and whipped cream, and then set. The fruit and whipped cream mixture is initially obtained by whipping 3.785 liters of cream. Later, it is intensely mixed with 3.785–5.67 liters of dried fruit, to which 453.6 grams of sugar are added.

Frozen Malt Products: To prepare frozen malt products, 13.24 liters of low-fat ice cream mix, 0.946 liters of malt syrup, a quantity of chocolate syrup obtained from 225 grams of cocoa (or 453.6 grams of chocolate syrup), 340.2 grams of sugar, and 0.946–1.419 liters of water are mixed and frozen.

Lactose-Free or Low-Lactose Ice Cream: Many consumers cannot fully digest lactose. Lactose malabsorption is sometimes accompanied by discomfort in the digestive system. In this condition, lactose is not digested in the small intestine and is fermented and produces gas and acid upon reaching the large intestine. Gas production causes pain and discomfort and can lead to diarrhea in acute cases. Often, individuals with lactose malabsorption can consume ice cream as part of a meal. The solution for individuals with more severe malabsorption is to consume lactose-free frozen desserts. These products are prepared from milk that has passed through ultrafiltration or diafiltration to remove lactose, or from milk in which lactose has been hydrolyzed. Ultrafiltration for lactose removal reduces the concentration of solids in the solution and increases the freezing point. On the other hand, lactose hydrolysis results in two glucose and galactose molecules for each lactose molecule, lowering the freezing point. By ultrafiltration and removing 50% of the lactose, and hydrolyzing the remaining lactose, the initial freezing point is maintained. It should be noted that all methods of lactose reduction definitely come with increased ice cream production costs.

Smoothies: Smoothies are beverages made by blending fresh or frozen fruit, fruit juice, and frozen milkshake mix, yoghurt, or sherbet. They fall into a category similar to milkshakes but often feature a broader range of flavoring ingredients. While various formulations exist for smoothies, a typical recipe includes a combination of whole fruit and/or fruit juice, cream or yoghurt, and crushed ice. This mixture is blended using a high-speed blender and served promptly.

Drinkable Probiotic Ice Cream (Milkshakes): Milkshakes are typically prepared for immediate consumption at retail outlets, often fast-food establishments. These shakes are made using milkshake mixes produced at dairy processing facilities, which are then packaged and shipped in bulk containers. A typical milkshake mix contains approximately 3% milk fat, 13% milk solids-not-fat, 8% sugar, 3% corn syrup solids, and 0.4% stabilizer, resulting in a total solids content of around 28.4%. Milkshakes can also be crafted in ice cream retail shops by blending scooped ice cream with milk using a high-speed blender, following a more traditional approach than using a freezing machine (Marshall et al. 2003; Homayouni 2008).

References

Homayouni, A. (2008). Effect of microencapsulation and resistant starch on the probiotic survival and sensory properties of synbiotic ice cream. PhD thesis. University of Tehran, Iran.

Marshall, R.T., Goff, H.D., and Hartel, R.W. (2003). *Ice Cream*, 6e. New York: Kluwer Academic/Plenum Publishers 371 pp.

2

Probiotics: Definition and Characterization

2.1 Introduction

The number of microbial cells in the gut is ten times greater than the number of cells that make up an adult's body. Therefore, the alteration of the gut microbial balance affects the host's health. In this context, the greater the proportion of beneficial microbes (probiotics) compared to harmful microbes, the host experiences better health and is less susceptible to diseases. One way to maintain a high number of beneficial microbes in the gut is by introducing probiotics into the gut through regular consumption of foods containing these microbes. Among various food types, dairy products, especially yoghurt, have the capability to effectively deliver probiotics to the human intestine. Since probiotic cells need to reach the gut alive to establish residency, grow, reproduce, and exert health-promoting effects, the question arises: How can probiotic cells be successfully delivered and remain alive in the gut? What role do environmental factors such as production, storage, consumption conditions (high sucrose concentration, presence or absence of oxygen, low freezing temperature, and preservation) of ice cream, as well as internal factors such as gastric acid and initial intestinal alkalinity, play in the viability of probiotics?

On the other hand, it has been shown that certain carbohydrates, which are not fully digested and absorbed in the small intestine, reach the large intestine undigested and provide nourishment for probiotics. These compounds, known as prebiotics, serve as a carbon and energy source for probiotics. Prebiotics can be used in the formulation of ice cream. A food product that contains both probiotic and prebiotic components is called a synbiotic. Synbiotic foods are classified as beneficial foods. In recent years, the technology of encapsulating probiotics in edible coatings for the physical protection of these cells against adverse production, storage,

Probiotic Ice Cream: Science and Technology, First Edition. Aziz Homayouni-Rad.

distribution, and consumption conditions during the shelf life of ice cream has gained attention. The health-promoting effects of probiotics result from the activities of live cells, dead cells, cell walls, cytoplasmic components, and their metabolites in the digestive system. As previously mentioned, the indicator of probiotic properties is the bacterial activity and performance under physiological conditions (gastrointestinal tract). There are three methods to increase and maintain the population of probiotics and enhance their beneficial effects in the gut, including the consumption of probiotics through various food and pharmaceutical products, the intake of prebiotic compounds along with food, and avoiding factors that reduce probiotic populations in the gut, such as an unhealthy diet, radiation, stress, illness, and drugs. Therefore, the health benefits of probiotics encompass both preventive and therapeutic aspects (nutrition and medicine). The preventive and therapeutic use of probiotics has several advantages compared to antibiotics. These include avoiding the harmful side effects of antibiotics, such as the elimination of beneficial gut flora, which weakens the immune system and increases the risk of infectious diseases and allergies. Additionally, the risk of bacterial resistance to antibiotics increases. Today, probiotic products have gained considerable acceptance, with around products containing *Lactobacillus acidophilus* and *Bifidobacterium bifidum* being produced worldwide. In 1993, more than probiotic dairy products were consumed publicly in Japan. Examples of probiotic dairy products include ice cream, frozen dairy desserts, kefir, buttermilk, yoghurt, cheese, sour cream, cultured butter, cultured cream, infant food, water-based dairy beverages, and fermented milk with various flavors. The health-promoting effects of probiotics include the following (Homayouni 2008):

1. They have antimutagenic and anticarcinogenic effects.
2. They strengthen and stimulate the body's immune system.
3. They have anti-infectious effects.
4. They reduce serum cholesterol levels.
5. They improve lactose intolerance.
6. They enhance nutritional value by synthesizing vitamins (B and K) and improving the absorption of minerals like calcium, iron, zinc, manganese, copper, and phosphorus.
7. They reduce the likelihood of allergies.
8. They alleviate constipation.
9. They lower blood pressure.
10. They reduce bloating and abdominal swelling.
11. They improve hepatitis condition.
12. They reduce the complications of liver disease.

2.2 Definition of Probiotics

The term "probiotic" is derived from the Greek root "probios," meaning for life. It is juxtaposed with "antibiotic," referring to substances that are against life. This term was initially used to describe compounds produced by protozoa to stimulate the growth of other protozoa. In the early 1970s, Sperti extended the concept of this term to refer to a trophic substance that stimulates the growth of microorganisms. Later, Parker applied this term to feed supplements that, through balancing the microbial load of the intestines, induce beneficial effects in animals. Subsequently, the term "probiotic" was used for microorganisms and their compounds that lead to the balance of gut microbial flora, although the definition was not precise due to the inclusion of potentially harmful microorganisms as well. Fuller corrected the definition of the term "probiotic" as follows: live microorganisms that, when consumed as a dietary supplement, beneficially affect the host's health by maintaining the balance of the gut microbiota. This description has evolved over the years. Today, the term refers to nonpathogenic live microorganisms (such as lactic acid bacteria and yeasts used in fermented products) that, when consumed alone or in combination at sufficient doses, improve host health by enhancing the ratio of beneficial bacteria in the gut. According to the latest definition, probiotics are microorganisms that, when ingested in sufficient quantities as live organisms, confer health benefits to the host. A microorganism can be considered a probiotic if it possesses the following four attributes:

1. Easily producible on an industrial scale.
2. Viability throughout food production and storage.
3. Tolerance to the host's gastrointestinal conditions.
4. Exhibits health-promoting effects on the host after consumption.

The viability of probiotics belonging to the *Bifidobacterium* and *Lactobacillus* genera can be enhanced by the use of prebiotic carbohydrates. A combination of probiotics and prebiotics, termed synbiotics, has therapeutic properties for certain gastrointestinal disorders. Most probiotic bacteria belong to the *Lactobacillus* and *Bifidobacterium* genera, but other microorganisms such as gram-positive cocci, Bacillus, yeasts, and certain strains of *Escherichia coli* have also been used as probiotics. Probiotic products are available in forms like powders, tablets, drinks, and probiotic dairy products. As shown in Figure 2.1, microbial safety is of paramount importance when selecting probiotics. Many lactic acid bacteria used in the fermentation of yoghurt, sauerkraut, and kefir, for example, have a historical record of human safety. *Lactobacilli* are generally recognized as safe

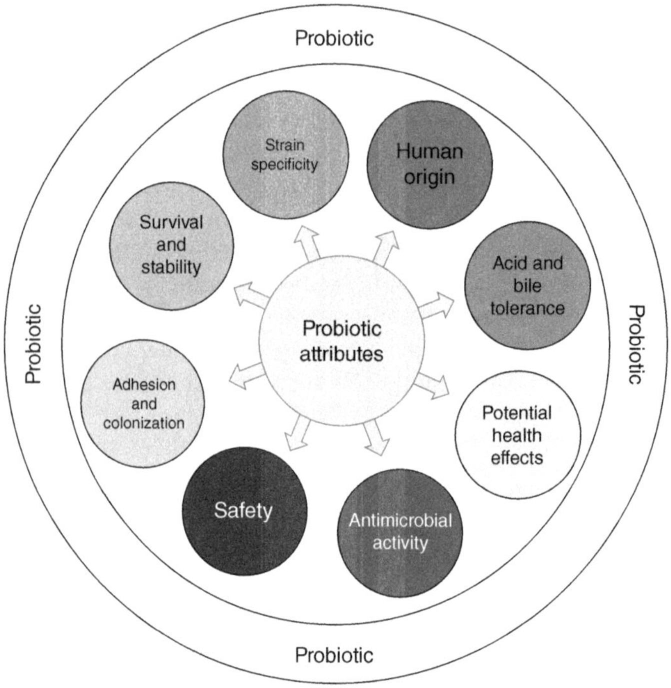

Figure 2.1 Desired characteristics for selecting suitable probiotic species.

(GRAS) due to their nonpathogenic nature. This holds true for certain species of *Bifidobacterium* as well. To determine the safety of a probiotic strain for humans, three stages of scientific research are conducted: initial in vitro and animal studies, controlled clinical trials with measurement of physiological factors, and consumption of the probiotic strain by humans over a period of time to gather data. One of the factors considered when selecting probiotic strains is their resistance to stressors originating from gastrointestinal conditions. For a probiotic strain to effectively reach its site of action (large intestine), it must survive the acidic conditions of the stomach and the alkaline secretions of the small intestine and must also compete with the existing gut microbiota. In vitro assays are considered simple methods for evaluating the resistance of probiotics to the mentioned conditions. However, sampling from the human stomach and small intestine is challenging and raises ethical concerns.

Another important factor in selecting probiotics is their resistance to antibiotics, which can be both an advantage and a drawback. While antibiotic resistance in probiotics can be advantageous when used for human treatment, the transfer of resistance genes from probiotic bacteria to pathogenic bacteria in the gut could render them resistant to drugs. For example, *Lactobacilli* and *Enterococci* can transfer antibiotic resistance genes to other bacteria through plasmids. Therefore, transferring resistance genes to other microorganisms might render some drugs ineffective. Another crucial characteristic in probiotic selection is their ability to adhere to intestinal epithelial cells. In many cases, probiotic cells are washed out of the gastrointestinal tract and excreted, such that one week after cessation of probiotic consumption, they are no longer detectable in feces. To assess the adhesion ability of probiotics to intestinal cells, co-culturing with tissue (epithelial cells) and probiotic cells is examined. Research has shown that *Lactobacilli* tend to adhere more to intestinal cells than *Bifidobacteria*. The resistance of probiotics to stresses caused by food conditions during production and storage is also a significant consideration when selecting suitable probiotic species. With the International Dairy Federation stipulating the presence of 10^7 live bacteria per gram of dairy product at the time of consumption, extensive research is underway to identify appropriate probiotic species for each food product. To achieve this, probiotics are subjected to simulated or real food conditions. Resistance to low pH in various fermented products, presence of oxygen, refrigeration or freezing temperatures during storage, and more, are considered indicators for selecting suitable probiotics for these types of foods. The method of incorporating probiotics into food and ensuring their viability in the food matrix is crucial for their successful transfer from food to the gut. Dairy products not only supply viable probiotics but also promote the growth of *Bifidobacterium* species. For example, probiotics can remain viable in skim milk stored at 4°C for up to four weeks. Adding various oligosaccharides can further enhance their viability. Considering issues related to the viability of probiotics in food, such as creating anaerobic conditions and preventing secondary contamination, as well as unfavorable stomach and initial intestinal conditions for probiotics, research is focused on providing new solutions. Utilizing specific food components (prebiotics) that reach beneficial gut microorganisms (probiotics) is deemed a promising approach to addressing probiotic viability issues. Probiotic bacteria are capable of producing various metabolites that influence flavor, color, and texture of food. Among these compounds, lactic acid, acetic acid, propionic acid, hydrogen peroxide, carbon dioxide, diacetyl, acetaldehyde, short-chain fatty acids, nisin, acidolin, and acidophilin exhibit antimicrobial effects. These effects become crucial during the shelf life of stored food products and after their consumption in the human gastrointestinal tract. Production of antimicrobial compounds is considered a prominent characteristic of probiotic bacteria. Moreover, various carbohydrate compounds like dextran, produced by lactic acid bacteria during fermentation and secreted outside bacterial cells, increase the viscosity of food materials. Antimicrobial compounds from probiotic bacteria exhibit inhibitory effects on microorganisms such as *Clostridium perfringens*, *Clostridium difficile*, *Clostridium tyrobutyricum*, *E. coli*, *Salmonella typhimurium*, Enterobacter species, *Listeria monocytogenes*, *Bacillus cereus*, and *Staphylococcus aureus*. Organic acids and low molecular weight peptides produced by *Lactobacillus casei* and acidolin from *L. acidophilus*, are capable of inhibiting *E. coli* and *Streptococcus mutans*. *L. acidophilus* produces the highest level of antimicrobial compounds in fermented dairy products (Homayouni 2009).

2.3 Types of Probiotics

The general definition of probiotics as live microorganisms that have beneficial health effects on humans has made their identification and nomenclature challenging. The classification of probiotics in the past and present has been associated with errors. For example, in the past, it was believed that *Lactobacillus* GG belonged to the *L. acidophilus* genus. However, species of *L. acidophilus* cannot ferment pentoses (five-carbon sugars), and the final product of glucose fermentation by this bacterium is lactic acid (DL). In contrast, *Lactobacillus* GG ferments pentoses and produces L-lactic acid. This behavior is similar to *Lactobacillus rhamnosus* species. Today, *Lactobacillus* GG is classified as a bio-type of the nonlactose fermenting strains of *L. rhamnosus*. In general, most probiotic bacteria used in food, dietary supplements, and drugs are primarily from the lactic acid bacteria group, mainly belonging to the genera *Lactobacillus* and *Bifidobacterium*. However, other nonlactic acid bacteria such as *B. cereus toyoi*, *Bacillus clausii*, *Bacillus pumilus*, *E. coli Nissle*, *Propionibacterium freudenreichii*, *Propionibacterium jensenii*, *Propionibacterium acidopropionici*, *Propionibacterium thoenii*, and *Saccharomyces cerevisiae boulardii* are also often found as probiotics in the market. In Table 2.1, the most important probiotic species that are commonly used for human consumption are classified into four categories: lactic acid bacteria of the *Lactobacillus* genus, lactic acid bacteria of the *Bifidobacterium* genus, other lactic acid bacteria, and nonlactic acid bacteria. Since most probiotics belong to the genera *Lactobacillus* and *Bifidobacterium*, we will proceed to discuss their taxonomical, ecological, and growth requirements in the following sections (Homayouni 2009).

Table 2.1 Most important probiotic species for human consumption.

***Lactobacillus* species**	***Bifidobacterium* species**	**Other lactic acid bacteria**	**Nonlactic acid bacteria**
Lactobacillus acidophilus	*Bifidobacterium adolescentis*	*Enterococcus faecalis*	*Bacillus cereus toyoi*
Lactobacillus amylovotus (L. casei)	*Bifidobacterium animalis (lactis)*	*Enterococcus faecium*	*Escherichia coli Nissle*
Lactobacillus crispatus	*Bifidobacterium bifidum*	*Sporolactobacillus inulinus*	*Propionibacterium freudenreichii*
Lactobacillus delbrueckii subsp. bulgaricus	*Bifidobacterium breve*		*Saccharomyces cerevisiae boulardii*
Lactobacillus gallinaruma	*Bifidobacterium infantis*		
Lactobacillus gasseri	*Bifidobacterium longum*		
Lactobacillus johnsonii			
Lactobacillus paracasei			
Lactobacillus plantarum			
Lactobacillus reuteri			
Lactobacillus rhamnosus			

2.3.1 *Lactobacillus* Genus

The species belonging to the *Lactobacillus* genus are shown in Table 2.2. These bacteria were introduced as *Lactobacillus* in the 1986 edition of the book "Bergey's Manual." *L. acidophilus*, *Lactobacillus laxacius*, *Lactobacillus plantarum*, *L. casei*, and *Lactobacillus fermentum* are among the most important species residing in the human intestines. Among them, *L. acidophilus* has been primarily used in the production of probiotic foods. Bacteria of the *Lactobacillus* genus are Gram-positive, nonspore-forming, catalase-negative, and usually nonmotile. They are also resistant to salt and phage. *Lactobacilli* can be divided into two categories based on their glucose fermentation pattern: homofermentative (homogeneous fermentation) and heterofermentative (heterogeneous fermentation). Homofermentative

Table 2.2 Species belonging to the genus *Lactobacillus*.

Lactobacillus plantarum	*Lactobacillus jensenii*
Lactobacillus acetotolerans	*Lactobacillus reuteri*
Lactobacillus curvatus	*Lactobacillus johnsonii*
Lactobacillus acidophilus	*Lactobacillus rhamnosus*
Lactobacillus delbrueckii	*Lactobacillus kandleri*
Lactobacillus agilis	*Lactobacillus ruminis*
Lactobacillus farciminis	*Lactobacillus kefir*
Lactobacillus alimentarius	*Lactobacillus kefiranofaciens*
Lactobacillus fermentum	*Lactobacillus salivarius*
Lactobacillus amylophilus	*Lactobacillus mali*
Lactobacillus fructivorans	*Lactobacillus sanfrancisco*
Lactobacillus amylovorus	*Lactobacillus sharpe*
Lactobacillus fructosus	*Lactobacillus suebicus*
Lactobacillus avarius	*Lactobacillus vaccinostercus*
Lactobacillus gallinarum	*Lactobacillus vaginalis*
Lactobacillus bifermentans	*Lactobacillus viridescens*
Lactobacillus gasseri	*Lactobacillus crispatus*
Lactobacillus graminis	*Lactobacillus intestinalis*
Lactobacillus buchneri	*Lactobacillus pontis*
Lactobacillus halotolerans	*Lactobacillus sake*
Lactobacillus casei subspecies casei	*Lactobacillus malefermentans*
Lactobacillus hamsteri	*Lactobacillus minor*
Lactobacillus collinoides	*Lactobacillus suebicus*
Lactobacillus helveticus	*Lactobacillus murinus*
Lactobacillus confusus	*Lactobacillus orisa*
Lactobacillus hilgardii	*Lactobacillus parabuchneri*
Lactobacillus coryniformis	*Lactobacillus paracasei*
Lactobacillus homohiochii	*Lactobacillus pentosus*

lactobacilli ferment glucose via the glycolytic pathway, converting one molecule of glucose into two molecules of pyruvate, and eventually into two molecules of lactic acid, along with two molecules of ATP. Examples of obligatory homofermentative *lactobacilli* include *L. acidophilus, Lactobacillus crispatus, Lactobacillus gallinarum, Lactobacillus gasseri*. Heterofermentative *lactobacilli*, on the other hand, ferment glucose through the pentose phosphate pathway, producing lactate, carbon dioxide, ethanol, and one molecule of ATP. These bacteria also produce one molecule each of pentose and lactate during fermentation. Obligatory heterofermentative *lactobacilli* include *L. fermentum* and *Lactobacillus reuteri*. Furthermore, *L. casei*, *Lactobacillus paracasei subsp. paracasei*, *L. paracasei subsp. tolerance*, and *L. plantarum* are considered facultative heterofermentative *lactobacilli*. Overall, *Lactobacillus* species play a significant role in human and animal gut microbiota and are widely used in probiotic applications due to their beneficial properties (Homayouni 2009).

2.3.1.1 *Lactobacillus acidophilus*

L. acidophilus is mostly found in the human and animal small intestines and urinary tract. This bacterium possesses beta-galactosidase activity and is more resistant to gastric acid and bile salts compared to *L. casei*, *L. paracasei*, *L. rhamnosus*, and *B. bifidum*. It does not produce a double layer of bile salts more than the mentioned species. *L. acidophilus* is a Gram-positive, rod-shaped, nonspore-forming, homofermentative, and nonmotile bacterium. The lactic acid produced by it is in the form of a racemic mixture (D- and L-isomers), and it depends on environmental temperature. It produces L-lactic(+) acid at 45°C and L-lactic(−) acid at 10°C. Nutritionally, this bacterium is auxotrophic, requiring organic nitrogen sources (free amino acids and small peptides) and B-group vitamins. Its optimal growth temperature is between 35 and 40°C, and it does not grow well at refrigeration temperatures. The optimal pH for its growth is 5.5–6, and growth is inhibited below pH 4. *L. acidophilus* grows slowly in milk and has a low acid-producing rate. It is sensitive to yoghurt conditions and tends to disappear rapidly during yoghurt storage. Other characteristics of *L. acidophilus* include halotrophic, microaerophilic, better growth in the presence of 5–10% carbon dioxide gas, and the ability to ferment amygdalin and various sugars, including sucrose, fructose, galactose, glucose, lactose, maltose, mannose, sucrose, and trehalose. This bacterium produces metabolites from lactose and nitrogen-containing compounds (such as the amino acid threonine), as well as producing acetaldehyde. Morphologically, its cells are observed in single, paired, or chain forms. Sometimes, the clustering of cell chains results in clumps resembling bunches. The colonies of these bacteria appear cream-colored and circular (on the bottom surface of culture media), triangular and convex lens-shaped (in the thickness of the culture media).

2.3.1.2 *Lactobacillus casei*

L. casei is another of the most important probiotic species that has found widespread use in food products. In the industry, this bacterium is used for producing lactic acid from whey. *L. casei* also resides in the human small intestine. It has good resistance to gastric acid and bile salts. *L. casei* is a Gram-positive, rod-shaped, nonspore-forming, heterofermentative, and nonmotile bacterium. The lactic acid produced by this species is of the L-form(+). *L. casei* displays good resistance against Vancomycin. It has better survivability in dairy products compared to other species. Morphologically, cells of *L. casei* are observed in single, paired, or short-chain forms. Colonies of this bacterium also appear cream-colored. In deeper layers of the culture medium, they are seen as circular with a faint halo, while in the thicker parts of the medium, they present a triangular shape (Homayouni 2009).

2.3.2 Genus *Bifidobacterium*

The species belonging to the genus *Bifidobacterium* are shown in Table 2.3. These bacteria were introduced in the 1986 edition of the book "*Bifidobacterium*" by Foundations Press. The species of *Bifidobacterium* (*B. bifidum*, *Bifidobacterium longum*, *Bifidobacterium infantis*, *Bifidobacterium breve*, *Bifidobacterium adolescentis*, *Bifidobacterium angulatum*, *Bifidobacterium catenulatum*, *Bifidobacterium dentium*, and *Bifidobacterium pseudocatenulatum*) are inhabitants of the human large

Table 2.3 *Bifidobacterium* genus species.

Bifidobacterium adolescentis	*Bifidobacterium pseudolongum*
Bifidobacterium indicum	*Bifidobacterium choerinum*
Bifidobacterium angulatum	*Bifidobacterium pullorum*
Bifidobacterium infantis	*Bifidobacterium coryneform*
Bifidobacterium animalis (lactis)	*Bifidobacterium ruminantium*
Bifidobacterium longum	*Bifidobacterium cuniculi*
Bifidobacterium asteroides	*Bifidobacterium saeculare*
Bifidobacterium magnum	*Bifidobacterium dentium*
Bifidobacterium bifidum	*Bifidobacterium subtile*
Bifidobacterium merycicum	*Bifidobacterium gallicum*
Bifidobacterium boum	*Bifidobacterium suis*
Bifidobacterium minimum	*Bifidobacterium gallinarum*
Bifidobacterium breve	*Bifidobacterium thermophilum*
Bifidobacterium pseudocatenulatum	*Bifidobacterium globosum*
Bifidobacterium catenulatum	

intestine. Among these, *B. longum* has the highest population of *Bifidobacterium* species in the human colon. Other *Bifidobacterium* species can be isolated from the human reproductive tract, decayed teeth, fecal matter, and fermented milks. As *B. bifidum (Bb12)* has been isolated from the feces of healthy adults, it is often used in the production of dairy and nondairy probiotic products (Homayouni 2009).

Bifidobacterium bacteria are Gram-positive, nonspore-forming, catalase-negative, urease-positive, and usually nonmotile organisms. Their shape is often short rod-like, which can change based on the nutritional conditions of the growth environment. The optimal pH range for their growth is 6.5–7, and their optimal growth temperature is typically between 37 and 41°C. They are highly sensitive to acidity and are obligate anaerobes, meaning molecular oxygen is toxic to them. *Bifidobacteria* ferment sugars through the fructose-6-phosphate pathway and the bifidus shunt. The key enzyme in these reactions is fructose-6-phosphate phosphoketolase, which converts fructose-6-phosphate into acetyl-1-phosphate and erythrose-4-phosphate, and subsequently, erythrose-4-phosphate is converted to pyruvate. This biochemical reaction yields three moles of acetate and two moles of lactate. In terms of glucose fermentation pattern, they exhibit heterofermentation. The products of fermenting two moles of hexose sugars (six-carbon sugars) are three moles of acetate and two moles of lactate. The produced lactic acid by these bacteria is of the L(+) type. Additionally, small amounts of formic acid and gluconate are also produced. *Bifidobacteria* are capable of fermenting glucose and galactose. Some are even capable of breaking down D-galactosamine, D-glucosamine, amylose, and amylopectin. These characteristics are used for the identification of these bacteria. *Bifidobacteria* are saccharolytic bacteria (fermenting sugars). Therefore, milk is not a suitable medium for their growth. They often have higher nutritional requirements and rely on nonprotein organic nitrogen and B-group vitamins for growth. *Bifidobacteria* tend to have greater adhesive properties to intestinal epithelial cells compared to *L. acidophilus*. They are usually resistant to antimicrobials such as Nalidixic acid, Neomycine, Polymyxin B, and Metronidazole. However, they are sensitive to Vancomycin. Morphologically, *Bifidobacterium* cells appear as short rod-like, solitary, or clustered structures. Colonies of these bacteria appear as round, black colonies on the surface of culture media (unlike *L. acidophilus*). In thicker cultures, lentil-shaped colonies can also form (Homayouni 2009).

2.3.2.1 *Bifidobacterium lactis*

Bifidobacterium lactis (animalis) is often used in fermented dairy products. It exhibits greater resistance to oxygen and acidity compared to other species.

2.3.2.2 *Bifidobacterium longum*

B. longum is now commonly used in fermented dairy products. The species *B. longum* is capable of fermenting arabinogalactan, arabic gum, and tragacanth. *B. longum* and *B. infantis* exhibit the highest adhesion capability to intestinal cells.

2.3.3 Other Lactic Acid Bacteria

Some lactic acid bacteria belonging to other genera, such as *Enterococcus faecalis*, *Enterococcus faecium*, and *Sporolactobacillus inulinus*, are also classified as probiotics.

2.3.4 Nonlactic Acid Bacteria Probiotics

The probiotic properties of certain nonlactic acid bacteria, such as *B. cereus* (Toyoi), *E. coli (Nissle)*, and *P. freudenreichii*, have been established.

2.3.5 Probiotic Yeasts

It has been shown that certain yeasts, such as *Saccharomyces cerevisiae var. boulardii*, possess probiotic properties.

2.4 Health-Promoting Effects of Probiotics

Probiotics are types of microorganisms that reside beneficially in the human digestive system and have various impacts on health. These effects include the following:

1. **Gut Microbiome Balance:** Probiotics contribute to maintaining a balanced gut microbiome. This balance is crucial for various aspects of health, including digestion, immune function, and overall well-being.
2. **Digestive Health:** Probiotics can help improve digestive health by promoting the growth of beneficial bacteria, preventing the overgrowth of harmful bacteria, and enhancing the overall functioning of the digestive system.
3. **Immune System Support:** Probiotics play a role in supporting the immune system. They can help modulate immune responses and enhance the body's defenses against infections and illnesses.
4. **Gastrointestinal Disorders:** Probiotics have been studied for their potential to alleviate symptoms of gastrointestinal disorders such as

irritable bowel syndrome (IBS), inflammatory bowel disease (IBD), and diarrhea.

5. **Nutrient Absorption:** Some probiotics aid in the absorption of nutrients, such as vitamins and minerals, by enhancing the gut's ability to break down and assimilate these nutrients.
6. **Mood and Mental Health:** Emerging research suggests a connection between the gut and the brain, known as the gut-brain axis. Probiotics may influence mood and mental health by affecting this axis.
7. **Reduced Antibiotic-Associated Side Effects:** Probiotics can help mitigate the side effects of antibiotics, such as antibiotic-associated diarrhea, by maintaining gut balance during antibiotic treatment.
8. **Oral Health:** Certain probiotics can contribute to oral health by inhibiting the growth of harmful bacteria in the mouth and reducing the risk of dental issues.
9. **Women's Health:** Probiotics can have positive effects on women's health, including maintaining vaginal health and preventing vaginal infections.
10. **Allergies and Atopic Conditions:** Some research suggests that probiotics might play a role in reducing the risk of allergies and atopic conditions by modulating the immune response.

It is important to note that the effects of probiotics can vary based on the specific strains used, the individual's health condition, and other factors. Consulting a healthcare professional is recommended before starting any probiotic regimen, especially for individuals with underlying health issues.

2.5 Necessity of Formulating Probiotic Ice Creams

Dairy products play a significant role in human health and constitute a major part of the dietary pyramid. The health-promoting and therapeutic effects of fermented dairy products have been utilized for many years. Nowadays, such foods are referred to as "beneficial" due to their nutritional value as well as their health-promoting and disease-preventive effects. In recent years, probiotics have been employed to enhance the health-promoting effects of dairy products. Probiotics are beneficial bacteria found in the human intestines. They constitute a significant portion of the gut bacteria and play a vital role in human health. Their primary function is to regulate the gut microbiota and enhance resistance against intestinal pathogens. As age increases, the proportion of beneficial bacteria in the intestines decreases, while putrefactive bacteria and pathogens increase. Putrefactive bacteria threaten human health by producing toxic substances in the large intestine. Therefore, it is essential to maintain an initial (high) population of probiotic bacteria in the intestines throughout life and prevent their reduction. Regular consumption of dairy products containing probiotics is one way to achieve this goal. In general, probiotics are used to treat various human disorders such as lactose intolerance, diarrhea, food allergies, intestinal infections, constipation, hepatitis, bloating, colitis, gastric acidity, high blood cholesterol, and cancer. They are particularly effective in treating gastrointestinal disorders, such as mucosal damage, inflammation, and changes in gut permeability. The most widely accepted therapeutic use of probiotics is in individuals sensitive to lactose intolerance. Probiotic bacteria like *L. acidophilus* and *Bifidobacteria* assist in digesting the lactose present in fermented dairy products by producing β-galactosidase. The digestion of lactose within the intestines continues with the help of probiotics. Effective treatment occurs when dairy products contain a minimum of 10^7 probiotic bacteria per gram of the product (Homayouni 2008).

2.6 Challenges in Production, Preservation, and Consumption of Probiotic Ice Cream

The production, preservation, and consumption of dairy products containing probiotics face several challenges that can affect the viability of probiotic bacteria. For instance, the pH of fermented dairy products like yoghurt (usually between 4 and 4.5) and the alkaline conditions of the intestine (alkaline zone) are not suitable for probiotics. Additionally, refrigeration temperatures during storage are lower than the optimal growth temperature for probiotics. Metabolites produced by yoghurt bacteria also negatively impact the survival of probiotics. On the other hand, the presence of oxygen in the product can also affect the viability of *bifidobacteria*, as they belong to anaerobic microorganisms. Several methods are employed to enhance the viability of probiotics in dairy products, including the addition of growth promoters, stopping fermentation at pH levels above 5, lowering fermentation temperatures, increasing fermentation duration, low-temperature storage, buffering with concentrated protein whey (for yoghurt), and applying hydrostatic pressure. However, none of these methods has proven entirely successful on its own. An essential factor in maintaining probiotic viability is selecting species that are resistant to the production and consumption conditions of food. These selected species should tolerate low-pH yoghurt, stomach acidity, and alkaline intestinal conditions. Additionally, they should remain viable during low-temperature production and storage (as seen in frozen dairy desserts). High sucrose concentration and oxygen presence in frozen dairy desserts also affect probiotic viability. Therefore, probiotics need to maintain their viability during the product's shelf life. An alternative approach to enhance probiotic viability is to provide physical protection against unfavorable production, preservation, and consumption conditions. Microencapsulation involves creating a protective shell around the probiotic microorganisms, aiding in their survival. This method has been used to increase the viability of *Bifidobacterium pseudolongum* in a simulated stomach environment. Additionally, in frozen dairy desserts, this method is used to increase the viability of *Lactobacillus delbrueckii subsp. bulgaricus* and prevent sensory changes. Conditions for processing frozen dairy products, which influence probiotic viability, have received limited research attention. These conditions include low storage temperatures, high sugar concentrations, and oxygen presence. Since most dairy products are stored at low temperatures, and some like ice cream and frozen yoghurt are stored under freezing conditions, the effects of these temperatures on probiotic viability require further investigation. In sweetened dairy products like ice cream and frozen yoghurt, high sugar concentrations pose challenges. Furthermore, the presence of high levels of oxygen due to air incorporation negatively affects probiotic viability. Since oxygen is inevitable in the atmospheric air and microaerophilic or anaerobic properties of probiotics must be maintained, replacing nitrogen and carbon dioxide as a substitute for air is necessary. Studies on the viability of *L. acidophilus* and *B. bifidum* in ice cream have shown that this product has good potential for distributing these probiotics among consumers. Low-fat ice cream, compared to high-fat ice cream, provides better conditions for the viability of *L. acidophilus*, *L. paracasei*, and *B. lactis*. Ice cream facilitates the growth of probiotics in a large number and the possibility of maintaining their viability during storage. An investigation into the viability of *Lactobacillus johnsonii* in ice cream at two different sugar and fat levels and two different temperatures revealed that the population of *L. johnsonii* does not decrease during 8 months of refrigerated storage. It has also been shown that this probiotic has high resistance to alkaline conditions, antibiotics, and acidity (Homayouni 1386). Research conducted by Homayouni (2008) has thoroughly investigated the effects of processing conditions on the viability of probiotics in ice cream. Conditions such as low storage temperatures (4°C and −20°C), high sugar concentrations (10, 15, 20, and 25%), and oxygen scavenger compounds (such as vitamin C and cysteine) were studied in detail. Particularly, valuable studies have been conducted on the impact of these conditions on the viability of *L. casei* (Homayouni 1386). Additionally, the use of resistant starch as a prebiotic compound in ice cream formulation and its effects on probiotic viability and sensory characteristics of ice cream have been investigated (Homayouni et al. 2008). Resistant starch can be utilized both in ice cream formulation and in the structure of a danka membrane (containing *L. casei* and *B. lactis*). It is certain that producing such products can enhance product diversity, competitive power, and market dominance for factories (Homayouni 2008).

References

Homayouni, A. (2008). Effect of microencapsulation and resistant starch on the probiotic survival and sensory properties of synbiotic ice cream. PhD thesis. University of Tehran, Iran.

Homayouni, A. (2009). *Therapeutical Effects of Functional Probiotic, Prebiotic and Synbiotic Foods*. Tabriz, Iran: Tabriz University of Medical Sciences.

Homayouni, A., Azizi, A., Ehsani, M.R., and Yarmand, M.S. (2008). Effect of microencapsulation and resistant starch on the probiotic survival and sensory properties of synbiotic ice cream. *Food Chemistry* 111 (1): 50–55.

3

Selection of Appropriate Probiotic Strains for Use in Probiotic Ice Cream

3.1 Selection of Appropriate Probiotic Strains for Use in Probiotic Ice Cream

Over the past two decades, various studies have highlighted the effectiveness of ice cream as a carrier for delivering probiotic bacteria like *Lactobacillus acidophilus* and *Bifidobacterium bifidum* to the human gut. Frozen dairy products, including ice cream, create ideal conditions for probiotic bacteria to survive during production, distribution, and storage (Homayouni 2008).

Some noteworthy aspects and findings related to probiotic ice cream include:

1. **Probiotic Growth and Survival:** Ice cream provides favorable conditions for probiotic bacteria to grow and thrive in significant numbers while maintaining their viability during storage. Low-fat ice cream, in particular, offers a conducive environment for the survival of probiotic strains like *Lactobacillus acidophilus*, *Lactobacillus paracasei*, and *Bifidobacterium lactis*.
2. **pH Impact:** Dairy frozen desserts prepared from yoghurt may reduce the bioavailability of certain probiotic strains due to their low pH (less than 4.5), which simulates the gastric environment. In contrast, fermented ice cream with a pH range of 6.5–6.6 is more favorable for probiotic survival.
3. **Stability During Storage:** Several studies have shown that probiotic counts in ice cream remain relatively stable during storage. For example, *Lactobacillus johnsonii* in ice cream with different levels of sucrose and fat did not decrease over eight months of cold storage. Similarly, *Lactobacillus rhamnosus (GG)* in ice cream with varying sucrose and fat levels showed no significant change over one year of storage at different temperatures.

Probiotic Ice Cream: Science and Technology, First Edition. Aziz Homayouni-Rad.

4. **Influence of Ingredients:** Inulin, a prebiotic, has been demonstrated to enhance the survival of probiotics like *Lactobacillus acidophilus* and *Bifidobacterium lactis* in ice cream. The use of casein hydrolysate or cysteine has also been found to have a protective effect on *Bifidobacterium lactis*.
5. **Sensory Considerations:** While probiotics can be successfully incorporated into ice cream, sensory analysis has shown that the taste of ice cream fermented with probiotic bacteria may be less accepted compared to nonfermented ice cream.
6. **Strain Selection:** The choice of probiotic strains is crucial for their adaptation to ice cream conditions. Some strains are inherently more stable, while others may require specific measures to ensure their viability.
7. **Survival Mechanisms:** Enhanced expression of certain proteins, such as stress proteins, may improve the survival of probiotics in ice cream. Exposure to stresses like carbon starvation, cold shock, and oxidative stress prior to ice cream production can favor probiotic survival.
8. **Optimizing Ice Cream Mixture:** Altering the composition of the ice cream mixture can enhance probiotic stability. Ingredients like inulin and antioxidants, along with the choice of probiotic strains, can play a significant role.

In summary, ice cream has been demonstrated to be a viable carrier for probiotic bacteria, with specific conditions and ingredient choices influencing probiotic survival and effectiveness. The selection of suitable probiotic strains and optimizing the ice cream formulation are critical factors in producing probiotic ice cream with desirable probiotic benefits.

3.2 Effect of pH on Growth and Viability of Probiotics in Culture Media

Since the primary aim of this research is to enhance the viability of probiotics throughout the stages of production, storage, and consumption of functional synbiotic ice cream, and considering that the digestive system and production conditions, such as freezing temperature, can have detrimental effects on probiotic microorganisms, it is logical to assess their viability under adverse process and consumption conditions before adding them to the final product. In doing so, the most resilient species among the available ones can be selected for incorporation into probiotic ice cream. To this end, several critical factors affecting the viability of probiotics during the process, storage, and consumption were chosen among many, including gastrointestinal conditions, particularly the stomach's acidic environment, which is the most limiting factor, and adverse conditions within the product (resulting from high sucrose concentration-induced osmotic pressure, freezing temperature, and the presence of atmospheric oxygen) were simulated. On the other hand, as comprehensive information regarding the growth and viability of probiotic species in both acidic and alkaline environments was limited, and considering the range of pH changes from the mouth to the small intestine, four probiotic species, including *Lactobacillus acidophilus*, *Lactobacillus casei*, *Bifidobacterium lactis*, and *Bifidobacterium longum*, were exposed to simulated gastric (pH 3-2) and intestinal (pH 8-7) conditions as well as the temporary transit through the initial part of the small intestine, where a transient shift from an acidic to an alkaline state occurs (pH 6-4). The most resilient species were identified. Furthermore, to simulate ice cream conditions, the effects of various sucrose concentrations (10, 15, 20, and 25%), the presence or absence of oxygen (air injection to achieve 100% overrun factor), and low refrigeration temperature (4°C for ice cream mixture) and freezing temperature (−20°C during freezing and storage of the final product) on the viability and growth of these four species were examined. Finally, the most resilient species were determined, and for additional physical protection against adverse factors in food matrices, calcium alginate and resistant starch microencapsulation were applied. These encapsulated probiotics were then added to the probiotic ice cream, and the viability of these bacteria was assessed over six months of storage at a specified temperature of −20°C. The suitable probiotic species, in order to exert its beneficial effects on the gastrointestinal tract, should not only withstand the conditions of ice cream but also surpass the high acidity of the stomach. The pH of the gastrointestinal tract varies in different parts, and it may drop as low as two in the stomach. To assess the viability of probiotic species, including *Lactobacillus acidophilus*, *Lactobacillus casei*, *Bifidobacterium lactis*, and *Bifidobacterium longum*, these bacteria were exposed to various pH levels, different sucrose concentrations, different oxygen concentrations, and low temperatures. The results of investigating the effect of pH levels (2–8) on the growth index of four probiotic species indicated a statistically significant difference at the 1% significance level among the bacteria. In other words, the bacteria exhibited different growth rates in different pH conditions (Table 3.1). Comparisons of means using the Duncan method at the 1% significance level showed that the highest growth was observed in *Lactobacillus casei* in pH conditions 6 and 7. As seen in Table 3.1, there is a statistically significant difference at the 1% significance level among the 7 pH levels tested. In other words, different pH conditions had different effects on bacterial growth. The comparisons of means in this

Table 3.1 Comparison of mean growth index of four probiotic bacteria in acidic and alkaline conditions by spectrophotometry at 525 nm wavelength using Duncan's test at a 5% significance level ($p < 0.05$).

Bacterial species	pH level	Mean growth
Lactobacillus acidophilus	2	0.0253 (i)
	3	0.0483 (hi)
	4	0.0137 (i)
	5	1.1503 (c)
	6	1.2567 (c)
	7	0.91 (d)
	8	0.9933 (d)
Bifidobacterium lactis	2	0.0527 (hi)
	3	0.0067 (i)
	4	0.0290 (i)
	5	0.2363 (g)
	6	0.5873 (e)
	7	0.4187 (f)
	8	0.4923 (ef)
Lactobacillus casei	2	0.0003 (i)
	3	0.1307 (ghi)
	4	0.1377 (ghi)
	5	1.5413 (b)
	6	1.7347 (a)
	7	1.726 (a)
	8	1.6447 (ab)
Bifidobacterium longum	2	0 (i)
	3	0.0017 (i)
	4	0.0007 (i)
	5	0.1590 (ghi)
	6	0.8920 (d)
	7	0.5413 (ef)
	8	0.2130 (gh)

Note: Different letters indicate statistically significant differences.
Explanation:

- "i" denotes insignificant.
- Letters "a," "b," "c," "d," "e," "f," "g," "h," and "i" indicate statistically significant differences, with "a" representing the highest mean growth and "i" representing the lowest mean growth.

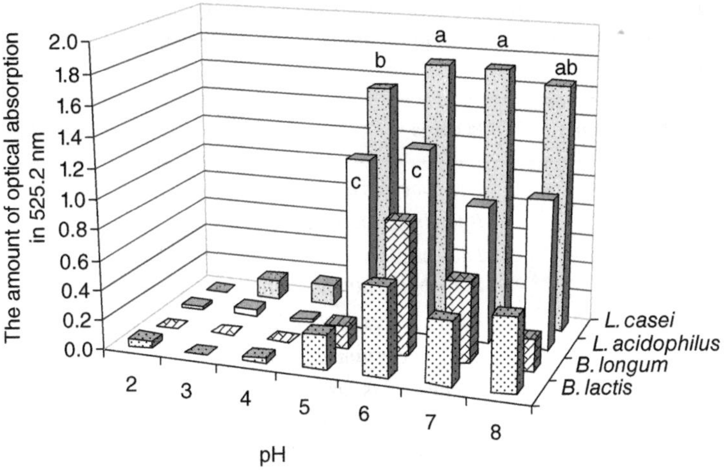

Figure 3.1 The effect of acidic and alkaline pH on the growth index of four probiotic bacteria.

regard using the Duncan method at the 1% significance level showed that the highest growth was for *Lactobacillus casei* in pH conditions 6 and 7. Additionally, there is a significant interaction effect at the 1% significance level between different pH levels and different bacteria. Therefore, it is not possible to compare the means between different pH levels and different bacteria and subsequently identify the best pH and bacteria. In these cases, a combination of treatments is compared to determine the best combination of bacteria and pH. Figure 3.1 shows that *Lactobacillus casei* exhibits the best growth in pH conditions 6 and 7. All probiotic species tested showed the lowest growth at pH 2 (Homayouni 2008).

The viability of these bacteria after three hours in pH 2 and 8 was examined. The experiment was conducted in a factorial design ($4 \times 3 \times 2$) using a complete randomized design, and the data were analyzed using SAS software. The results of studying the viability of these bacteria after three hours in pH 2 and 8 showed a statistically significant difference at the 1% significance level among the bacteria. In other words, the resistance of bacteria to different pH conditions was different. Comparisons of means in this regard using the Duncan method at the 1% significance level showed that the highest resistance was associated with *Lactobacillus casei* at pH = 8. As was seen in Table 3.2, there is a statistically significant difference at the 1% significance level between the two pH levels tested. In other words, different pH conditions had different effects on bacterial growth. The comparisons of means in this regard using the Duncan method at the 1% significance level showed that the highest growth was for *Lactobacillus casei* at pH = 8.

Table 3.2 Comparisons of mean viability index of four probiotic bacteria in acidic and alkaline conditions using spectrophotometry at 525 nm wavelength with Duncan test at a 5% significance level.

pH	Time (hours)	Bacteria	Mean viability
2	1	*Lactobacillus acidophilus*	0.236 p[a]
		Bifidobacterium lactis	0.248 o
		Lactobacillus casei	1.2353 d
		Bifidobacterium longum	0.031w
	2	*Lactobacillus acidophilus*	0.26 q
		Bifidobacterium lactis	0.174 q
		Lactobacillus casei	1.2027 e
		Bifidobacterium longum	0.038 v
	3	*Lactobacillus acidophilus*	0.315 m
		Bifidobacterium lactis	0.1313 t
		Lactobacillus casei	1.1003 f
		Bifidobacterium longum	0.0087 x
8	1	*Lactobacillus acidophilus*	0.36 l
		Bifidobacterium lactis	0.1573 s
		Lactobacillus casei	1.5917 c
		Bifidobacterium longum	0.5803 h
	2	*Lactobacillus acidophilus*	0.3687 j
		Bifidobacterium lactis	0.168 r
		Lactobacillus casei	1.5943 b
		Bifidobacterium longum	0.5273 i
	3	*Lactobacillus acidophilus*	0.368 k
		Bifidobacterium lactis	0.1203 u
		Lactobacillus casei	1.6147 a
		Bifidobacterium longum	0.6537 g

a) Different letters indicate a significant statistical difference.

Additionally, there is a significant interaction effect at the 1% significance level between different time periods (1, 2, and 3 hours). Comparisons of means in this regard using the Duncan method at the 1% significance level showed that the highest growth was associated with the first hour for *Lactobacillus casei*. There is also a significant mutual effect at the 1% significance level between different pH levels × bacteria, pH levels × time, and bacteria × time. Therefore, it is not possible to compare the means between different pH levels, bacteria, and time periods and subsequently identify the best pH, bacteria, and time. In these cases, a combination of treatments

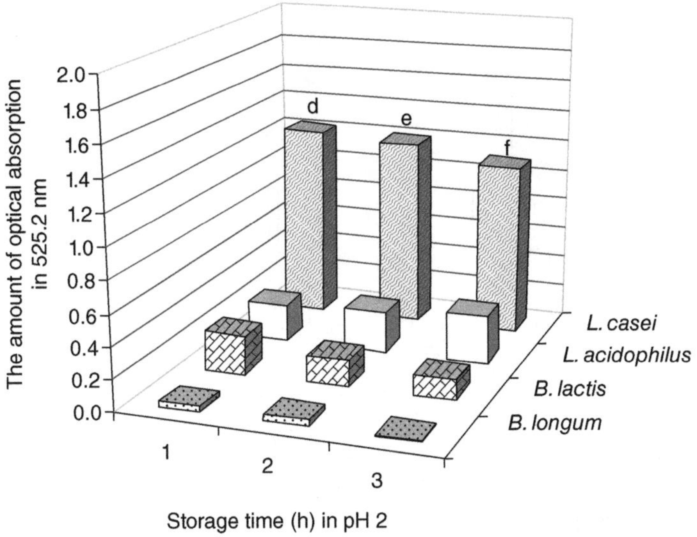

Figure 3.2 The effect of storage time on the viability of four probiotic species in pH = 2.

is compared to determine the best combination of pH × bacteria × time. The best combination of pH × bacteria was pH = 8 × *Lactobacillus casei*, the best combination of bacteria × time was *Lactobacillus casei* at one hour, and the best combination of pH × bacteria × time was *Lactobacillus casei* at pH = 8 and three hours (Figures 3.2 and 3.3).

The results showed that species belonging to the *Lactobacillus* genus exhibited greater relative resistance compared to the *Bifidobacterium* genus. This finding is consistent with previous research. It has been reported that *Lactobacillus* species in pH = 2 buffer decrease by about four logarithmic cycles, while *Bifidobacterium* species decrease by about five logarithmic cycles. However, the viability of bifidobacteria in low-pH environments depends on their specific species. Although some believe that a 90-minute duration is sufficient to study the viability of probiotics, this study considered a three-hour duration for the experiments and also excluded the effects of milk proteins and dairy products to examine the viability of probiotics under the most challenging conditions. Therefore, it is expected that species resistant to the conditions of this study would have better resistance in real conditions, such as dairy products and the digestive system. The high buffering capacity of milk proteins in dairy products enhances the viability of probiotics during their passage through the low-pH stomach. It has been reported that dairy products increase the

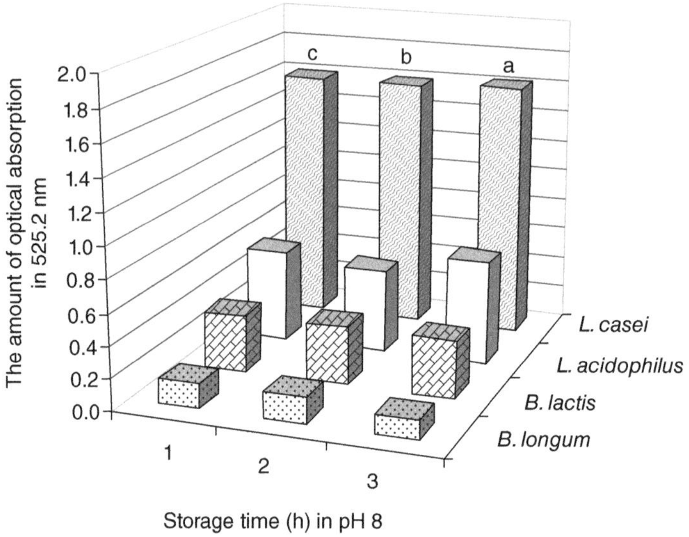

Figure 3.3 The effect of storage time on the viability of four probiotic species in pH = 8.

pH in the stomach by up to three units. Since the pH of most dairy products falls within the acidic range, and probiotics encounter acidic conditions in the stomach when consumed, the viability of probiotics in acidic conditions is of great importance compared to alkaline conditions. Therefore, viability in alkaline conditions alone is not valuable because the probiotic species may have already been lost before reaching alkaline conditions. On the other hand, acidic and alkaline conditions not only affect the growth and viability of probiotics but can also have mutual effects on their viability.

3.3 Effect of Different Sucrose Concentrations on the Growth and Viability of Bacteria in the Culture Medium

Some dairy products, such as ice cream, contain varying amounts of sugar (sucrose) in their formulations. The viability of probiotic strains used in these products may be influenced by osmotic pressure resulting from sucrose. In response to the question of how different sucrose concentrations (10, 15, 20, and 25%) affect the growth of four commercial probiotic strains, a factorial experiment (two factors 4 × 4) was conducted in a completely randomized design, and the obtained data were analyzed using SAS software. The results showed a significant difference between the bacteria at the 1% significance level, meaning that the bacteria had different growth

Table 3.3 Comparisons of mean growth index of four probiotic bacteria in different sucrose concentrations using spectrophotometry at a wavelength of 525 nm with Duncan test at a 5% significance level.

Sucrose (%)	Bacteria	Mean growth
10	*Lactobacillus acidophilus*	0.5607 c[a)]
	Bifidobacterium lactis	0.3827 d
	Lactobacillus casei	1.614 a
	Bifidobacterium longum	0.1167 efg
15	*Lactobacillus acidophilus*	0.5693 c
	Bifidobacterium lactis	0.26 de
	Lactobacillus casei	1.5043 ab
	Bifidobacterium longum	0.058 fg
20	*Lactobacillus acidophilus*	0.635 c
	Bifidobacterium lactis	0.204 def
	Lactobacillus casei	1.5413 a
	Bifidobacterium longum	0.0093 g
25	*Lactobacillus acidophilus*	0.6867 c
	Bifidobacterium lactis	0.0783 efg
	Lactobacillus casei	1.3387 b
	Bifidobacterium longum	0.0297 fg

a) Different letters indicate a significant statistical difference.

rates at different sucrose concentrations. The mean comparisons in this regard, using the Duncan method at the 1% significance level, revealed that the highest growth was related to *Lactobacillus casei* at sucrose concentrations of 10–20%. As shown in Table 3.3, there was a significant difference between the different sucrose concentrations at the 1% significance level, indicating that different sucrose concentrations had different effects on bacterial growth. The mean comparisons also showed that the highest growth was related to sucrose concentrations of 10–20% for *Lactobacillus casei*. Additionally, there was a significant interaction effect between different bacteria and sucrose concentrations at the 1% significance level. Therefore, instead of comparing the means using the Duncan method for different sucrose concentrations and four bacterial species, a two-factor treatment combination was compared. In the case of sucrose, the resistance of species belonging to the *Lactobacillus* genus was greater than that of species belonging to the *Bifidobacterium* genus. It has been shown that revival sugars such as maltose increase the growth and viability of probiotics like *Lactobacillus acidophilus*, *Lactobacillus reuteri*, and *Lactobacillus plantarum*. The results of this study indicated that although sucrose is not

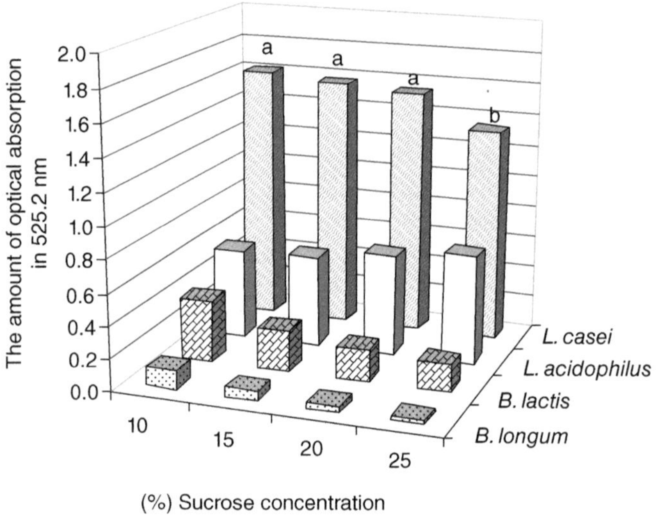

Figure 3.4 The effect of different sucrose concentrations on the growth index of four probiotic bacteria.

a revival sugar, it increased the growth of *Lactobacillus acidophilus* and *Lactobacillus casei* (Figure 3.4).

This table presents the mean growth index of four probiotic bacteria at different sucrose concentrations, analyzed using spectrophotometry at a wavelength of 525 nm with the Duncan test at a 5% significance level. The bacteria include *Lactobacillus acidophilus*, *Bifidobacterium lactis*, *Lactobacillus casei*, and *Bifidobacterium longum*. The table shows that different sucrose concentrations had different effects on the growth of these bacteria, and there were significant differences between the means. For example, *Lactobacillus casei* exhibited the highest growth in sucrose concentrations of 10 and 20%, while *Bifidobacterium longum* had the lowest growth at a sucrose concentration of 20%. The letters "a," "b," "c," "d," "e," "f," and "g" indicate significant differences between the means.

The viability of these bacteria was examined after three hours at different sucrose concentrations (10, 15, 20, and 25%). The experiment was conducted in a factorial design (three factors $4 \times 3 \times 4$) in a completely randomized design, and the obtained data were analyzed using SAS software. The results showed a significant difference between the bacteria at a one percent probability level. In other words, the resistance of bacteria to different sucrose concentrations varied. Mean comparisons in this regard using the Duncan method at a one percent probability level showed that the highest resistance was related to *Lactobacillus casei* at a 15% sucrose concentration. As seen in Table 3.4, there is a significant difference between

Table 3.4 Mean comparisons of viability index of four probiotic bacteria at different sucrose concentrations.

Sucrose (%)	Time (hours)	Bacteria	Mean viability
10	1	*Lactobacillus acidophilus*	0.704928 a14[a)]
		Bifidobacterium lactis	0.447026 a29
		Lactobacillus casei	1.651996 a7
		Bifidobacterium longum	0.01428 a47
	2	*Lactobacillus acidophilus*	0.62996 a18
		Bifidobacterium lactis	0.472931 a26
		Lactobacillus casei	1.85995 a1
		Bifidobacterium longum	0.008987 a48
	3	*Lactobacillus acidophilus*	0.502965 a1
		Bifidobacterium lactis	0.404623 a33
		Lactobacillus casei	0.721344 a4
		Bifidobacterium longum	0.027291 a43
15	1	*Lactobacillus acidophilus*	0.586909 a23
		Bifidobacterium lactis	0.461313 a28
		Lactobacillus casei	1.663548 a6
		Bifidobacterium longum	0.049908 a37
	2	*Lactobacillus acidophilus*	0.771587 a13
		Bifidobacterium lactis	0.420034 a31
		Lactobacillus casei	1.824661 a6
		Bifidobacterium longum	0.027989 a42
	3	*Lactobacillus acidophilus*	0.600005 a22
		Bifidobacterium lactis	0.39407 a34
		Lactobacillus casei	1.775556 a3
		Bifidobacterium longum	0.043015 a38
20	1	*Lactobacillus acidophilus*	0.612619 a21
		Bifidobacterium lactis	0.556367 a24
		Lactobacillus casei	1.629963 a8
		Bifidobacterium longum	0.042973 a39
	2	*Lactobacillus acidophilus*	0.676671 a16
		Bifidobacterium lactis	0.46567 a27
		Lactobacillus casei	0.579546 a12
		Bifidobacterium longum	0.037326 a40
	3	*Lactobacillus acidophilus*	0.621732 a20
		Bifidobacterium lactis	0.436921 a30
		Lactobacillus casei	1.664874 a5
		Bifidobacterium longum	0.031648a41

(Continued)

Table 3.4 (Continued)

Sucrose (%)	Time (hours)	Bacteria	Mean viability
25	1	*Lactobacillus acidophilus*	0.671252 a17
		Bifidobacterium lactis	0.420293 a32
		Lactobacillus casei	1.62435 a44
		Bifidobacterium longum	0.026309 a44
	2	*Lactobacillus acidophilus*	0.687738 a15
		Bifidobacterium lactis	0.376014 a35
		Lactobacillus casei	1.593906 a10
		Bifidobacterium longum	0.023994 a45
	3	*Lactobacillus acidophilus*	0.629008 a19
		Bifidobacterium lactis	0.335009 a36
		Lactobacillus casei	1.592896 a11
		Bifidobacterium longum	0.018989 a46

Note: The table compares the mean viability of four probiotic bacteria at different sucrose concentrations and different time intervals using the Duncan test at a 5% significance level.

a) Different a-numbers indicate a significant statistical difference.

the four sucrose levels at a one percent probability level. In other words, different sucrose concentrations had different effects on bacterial growth and survival. Mean comparisons in this regard using the Duncan method at a one percent probability level showed that the highest viability was related to a 15% concentration for *Lactobacillus casei*. Moreover, there is a significant difference between different time levels (1, 2, and 3 hours) at a one percent probability level. Mean comparisons in this regard using the Duncan method at a one percent probability level showed that the highest resistance was related to the two-hour period for *Lactobacillus casei*. Additionally, there is a significant interactive effect between different sucrose × bacteria levels, bacteria × time, and sucrose × time at a one percent probability level. Therefore, it is not possible to compare the mean levels of different sucrose, bacteria, and time, and accordingly introduce the best sucrose concentration, bacteria, and time. In these cases, a combination of treatments is compared to determine the best combination of sucrose, bacteria, and time. The best combination of sucrose × bacteria was 15% sucrose concentration with *Lactobacillus casei*. The best combination of bacteria × time was *Lactobacillus casei* at the two-hour time. The best combination of sucrose × time was 15% concentration at the two-hour time. And the best combination of sucrose × bacteria × time was *Lactobacillus casei* at 15% concentration and two hours (Figures 3.5–3.8). Alamprese and

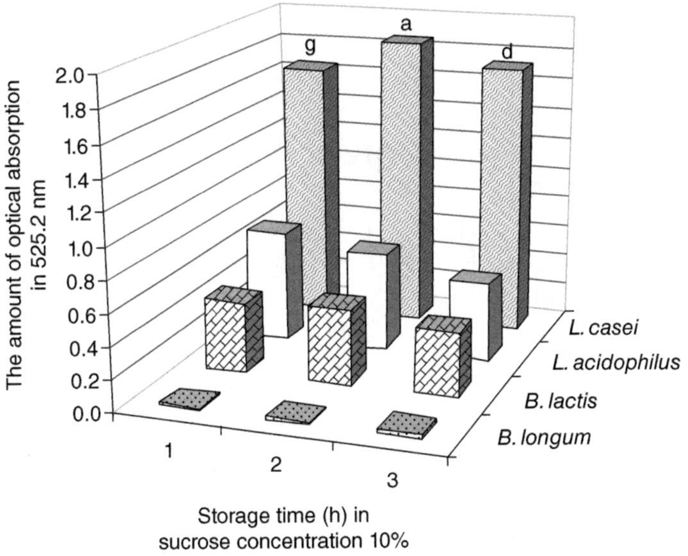

Figure 3.5 The effect of storage time in 10% sucrose on the viability index of four probiotic bacteria.

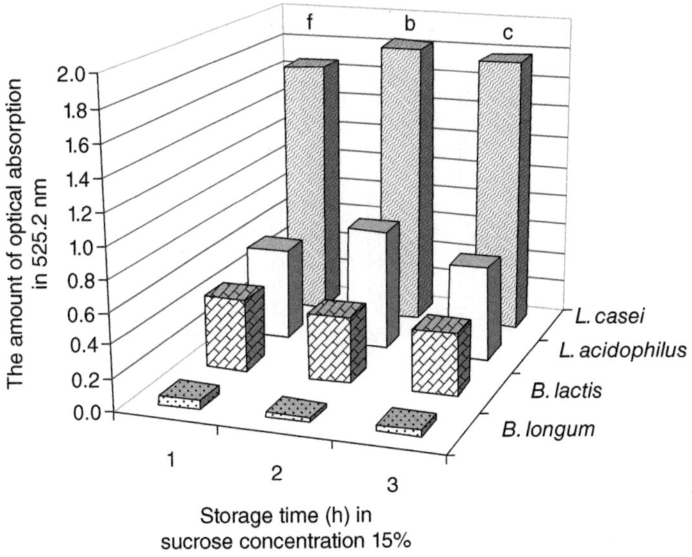

Figure 3.6 The effect of storage time in 15% sucrose on the viability index of four probiotic bacteria.

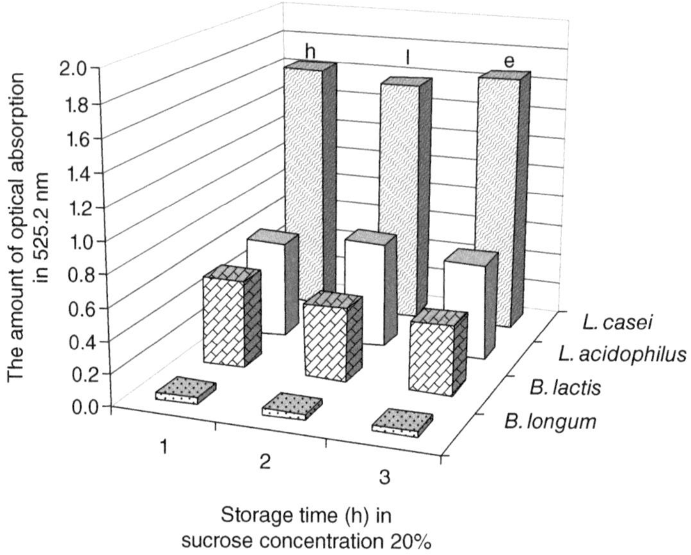

Figure 3.7 The effect of storage time in 20% sucrose on the viability index of four probiotic bacteria.

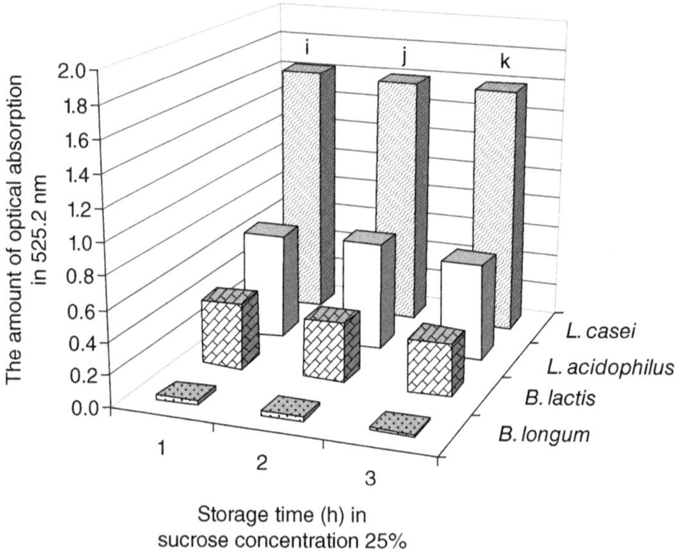

Figure 3.8 The effect of storage time in 25% sucrose on the viability index of four probiotic bacteria.

his colleagues also showed that sucrose concentrations of 15 and 17% in ice cream had no effect on the viability of *Lactobacillus johnsonii.*

3.4 Effect of Oxygen Scavengers on the Growth Index of Probiotics in the Culture Medium

In the freezing stage of ice cream production, air is injected into the product to the extent of the mixture's volume. Therefore, the expansion coefficient (overrun) of regular ice cream is approximately 100%. This means that the volume of the mixture doubles during freezing. Approximately, 21% of the air consists of oxygen gas. On the other hand, probiotic bacteria are often classified as anaerobic to microaerophilic, and molecular oxygen has a toxic and lethal effect on these bacteria. The use of oxygen-scavenging compounds such as ascorbic acid and packaging dairy products in oxygen-impermeable containers is one of the ways to reduce oxygen levels in these products. Ascorbic acid does not have much effect on the pH of dairy products but is capable of reducing the amount of oxygen and its potential for oxidation and revival. By reducing the amount of oxygen in the solution, the viability of probiotics increases. Hydrogen peroxide produced by lactic acid bacteria can also reduce the potential for oxidation and revival of dairy products. This action is associated with the absorption of free oxygen and the conversion of hydrogen peroxide to water. Adding cysteine and thiol-containing compounds to reduce the potential for oxidation and revival of the environment increases the growth and viability of probiotics. Furthermore, L-cysteine is an essential amino acid for probiotics and is used by probiotics as an amino-nitrogen compound. Since among probiotic bacteria, bifidobacteria are more fastidious than lactobacilli, adding cysteine seems necessary for the growth of these bacteria. The optimal amount of cysteine consumption, taking into account economic considerations and the viability of probiotics, is recommended to be 50 milligrams per liter of dairy product. However, the viability of *Lactobacillus rhamnosus* and *Lactobacillus paracasei* is not affected by cysteine. In this study, the effect of the presence or absence of air and the presence or absence of cysteine and vitamin C as oxygen-scavenging compounds in the culture medium on the growth index of four probiotic species was investigated. The results showed that cysteine had a positive effect on the growth of the tested species, and the growth of *Lactobacillus casei* in the presence of cysteine was higher than the other species. The effect of the oxygen content of the culture medium on the survival of probiotics depends on their species. The toxicity of oxygen to lactic acid bacteria may be an indirect effect in such a way that hydrogen peroxide is produced in the presence of oxygen by the flavoprotein oxidase enzyme present in lactic acid bacteria, which is considered a secondary metabolite. To investigate the effect of the presence or absence of air and oxygen-scavenging compounds on the growth index of four commercial probiotic species, the experiment was conducted in a factorial design (a three-factor, 4 × 2 × 3) in a completely randomized block design, and the obtained data were analyzed using SAS software. The results showed that cysteine had a significant effect on bacterial growth at a one percent level of probability. In other words, bacteria had different growth rates at different concentrations in the presence or absence of air and oxygen-scavenging compounds. Comparisons of means regarding the interaction effect of cysteine × vitamin C, using the Duncan test at a one percent level of probability, showed that cysteine had a positive effect on the growth of probiotics, while vitamin C had no effect on their growth. In this study, the highest growth was attributed to *Lactobacillus casei* in the culture medium containing cysteine (Table 3.5).

In this table, the mean growth index for four probiotic species is compared under different experimental conditions involving the presence of cysteine and vitamin C. The results show that cysteine had a positive effect on the growth of probiotics, while vitamin C had no significant impact on their growth. The interaction effect between cysteine and vitamin C was also found to be statistically significant. As shown in Table 3.6, the presence or absence of cysteine has a significant effect on the growth index of the four probiotic species at a one percent significance level. In other words, the presence of cysteine has a different effect compared to its absence. Comparisons of means using Duncan's test at a one percent significance level revealed that cysteine increases the growth index when compared to vitamin C. On the other hand, the presence or absence of air did not have a significant effect on the growth index of the bacteria. However, there was a significant interaction effect between bacterial species and the presence or absence of air at a one percent significance level. Comparisons

Table 3.5 Comparisons of mean growth index for four probiotic species in the presence of cysteine and vitamin C using spectrophotometry at a wavelength of 525.2 nm with Duncan's test at a 5% significance level.

Index experimental conditions	Mean growth		
Cysteine × vitamin C interaction effect	Cysteine	Control	Vitamin C
	0.8359 a[a)]	0.7429 b	0.7254 b

a) Different letters indicate statistically significant differences.

Table 3.6 Compares the mean interaction effect of cysteine, vitamin C, and the four probiotic bacterial species on growth index using spectrophotometry at a 5% significance level.

Oxygen absorber	Bacteria	Mean growth
Cysteine	*Lactobacillus acidophilus*	1.026 d[a]
	Bifidobacterium lactis	0.752 e
	Lactobacillus casei	1.5585 a
	Bifidobacterium longum	0.0072 g
Control	*Lactobacillus acidophilus*	1.1307 c
	Bifidobacterium lactis	0.3862 f
	Lactobacillus casei	1.4447 b
	Bifidobacterium longum	0.01g
Vitamin C	*Lactobacillus acidophilus*	1.05 d
	Bifidobacterium lactis	0.385 f
	Lactobacillus casei	1.4425 b
	Bifidobacterium longum	0.024 g

a) Different letters indicate a statistically significant difference.

of means in this regard showed that the highest growth was observed in *Lactobacillus casei* in an air-free culture medium. Additionally, there is a significant interaction effect between different bacterial species and the presence or absence of oxygen-absorbing compounds at a one percent significance level. Therefore, instead of comparing means in this case, the treatment combination of the two factors is considered. Table 3.7 shows that *Lactobacillus casei* has the highest growth in a culture medium containing cysteine. The interaction effect of bacterial species × presence or absence of air × presence or absence of oxygen-absorbing compounds is not significant. Our research results indicate that cysteine enhances the growth of *Lactobacillus casei* more than vitamin C (Figures 3.9 and 3.10). The addition of sodium bicarbonate can even further increase the growth of Lactobacillus and *Bifidobacterium* species compared to cysteine.

In this table, you can see the interaction effect of cysteine, vitamin C, and the four probiotic bacterial species on the growth index. The different letters indicate statistically significant differences between the groups. For example, the growth of *Lactobacillus casei* was significantly higher when cysteine was present compared to other conditions. The presence of vitamin C did not significantly affect the growth of these bacteria.

In this table, you can see the interaction effect of oxygen and the four probiotic bacterial species on the growth index. Different letters indicate

Table 3.7 Compares the mean interaction effect of oxygen and the four probiotic bacterial species on growth index using spectrophotometry at a 5% significance level.

With/without oxygen	Bacteria	Mean growth
With oxygen	*Lactobacillus acidophilus*	1.0817 c[a]
	Bifidobacterium lactis	0.5492 d
	Lactobacillus casei	1.4402 b
	Bifidobacterium longum	0.015 f
Without oxygen	*Lactobacillus acidophilus*	1.0561
	Bifidobacterium lactis	0.4662 e
	Lactobacillus casei	1.5236 a
	Bifidobacterium longum	0.0124 f

a) Different letters indicate a statistically significant difference.

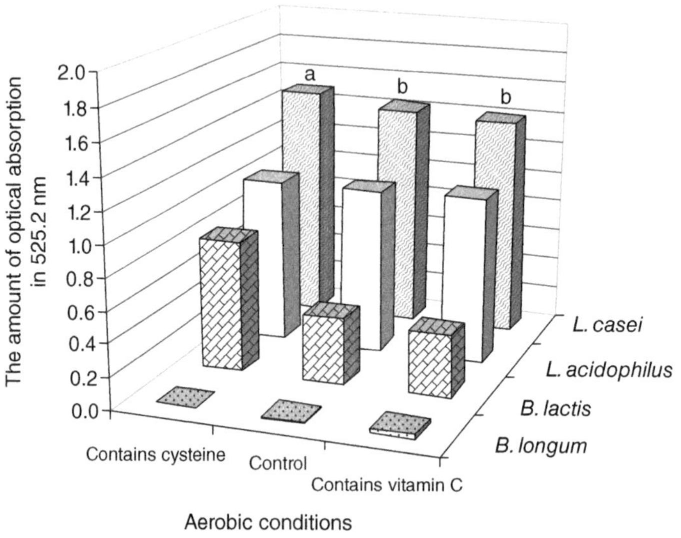

Figure 3.9 The effect of cysteine and vitamin C on the growth index of four probiotic bacteria in the presence of oxygen.

statistically significant differences between the groups. For example, the presence of oxygen significantly affected the growth of these bacteria, and different bacteria species responded differently to the presence or absence of oxygen.

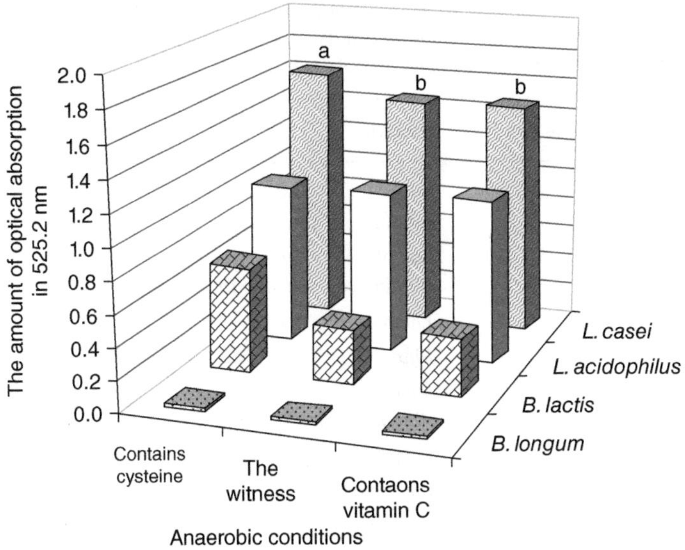

Figure 3.10 The effect of cysteine and vitamin C on the growth index of four probiotic bacteria in the absence of oxygen.

3.5 Effect of Different Processing Temperatures on the Viability Index of Probiotics in the Culture Medium

Probiotic bacteria, as part of dairy products, should be able to tolerate low temperatures (refrigerator and freezer). In this study, the effect of low temperatures (4 and −20°C) on the viability of four commercial probiotic species was examined over a period of three hours. The experiment was conducted in a factorial design (three factors: $4 \times 3 \times 2$) in a completely randomized design, and the data were analyzed using SAS software. The results showed a statistically significant difference between the bacteria at a one percent significance level. This means that the resistance of the bacteria to different temperatures was different (Table 3.8). Comparisons of means in this regard, using the Duncan method at a one percent significance level, showed that the highest resistance was related to *Lactobacillus casei* at −20°C. As shown in Table 3.8, there is a significant difference between the two temperature levels at a one percent significance level. Comparisons of means in this regard, using the Duncan method at a one percent significance level, showed that the highest viability was related to a temperature of −20°C for *Lactobacillus casei*. In other words, bacteria die

Table 3.8 Comparison of mean viability index of four probiotic bacteria at different temperatures over a three-hour period using spectrophotometry at a wavelength of 525.2 nm with Duncan test at a 5% significance level.

Temperature (°C)	Time (hours)	Bacteria	Mean viability
4	1	*Lactobacillus acidophilus*	1.2153 j[a)]
		Bifidobacterium lactis	0.5413 p
		Lactobacillus casei	1.4347 d
		Bifidobacterium longum	0.061 s
	2	*Lactobacillus acidophilus*	1.1757 1
		Bifidobacterium lactis	0.4547 q
		Lactobacillus casei	1.345 h
		Bifidobacterium longum	0.0323 x
	3	*Lactobacillus acidophilus*	1.2107 k
		Bifidobacterium lactis	0.665 n
		Lactobacillus casei	1.421 e
		Bifidobacterium longum	0.0563 t
−20	1	*Lactobacillus acidophilus*	1.2753 i
		Bifidobacterium lactis	0.5617 o
		Lactobacillus casei	1.488 a
		Bifidobacterium longum	0.0343 w
	2	*Lactobacillus acidophilus*	1.4167 f
		Bifidobacterium lactis	0.4373 r
		Lactobacillus casei	1.4843 b
		Bifidobacterium longum	0.0357 v
	3	*Lactobacillus acidophilus*	1.3848 g
		Bifidobacterium lactis	0.678 m
		Lactobacillus casei	1.4793 c
		Bifidobacterium longum	0.0387 u

a) Nonmatching letters indicate a statistically significant difference.

faster at temperatures close to freezing compared to lower temperatures. Furthermore, there is a significant difference between different time levels (1, 2, and 3 hours) at a one percent significance level. Comparisons of means in this regard, using the Duncan method at a one percent significance level, showed that the highest resistance was related to the first hour for *Lactobacillus casei*. Additionally, there is a significant interaction effect between temperature × bacteria, bacteria × time, and temperature × time at a one percent significance level. Therefore, it is not possible to compare the average levels between different temperature levels, bacteria, and times,

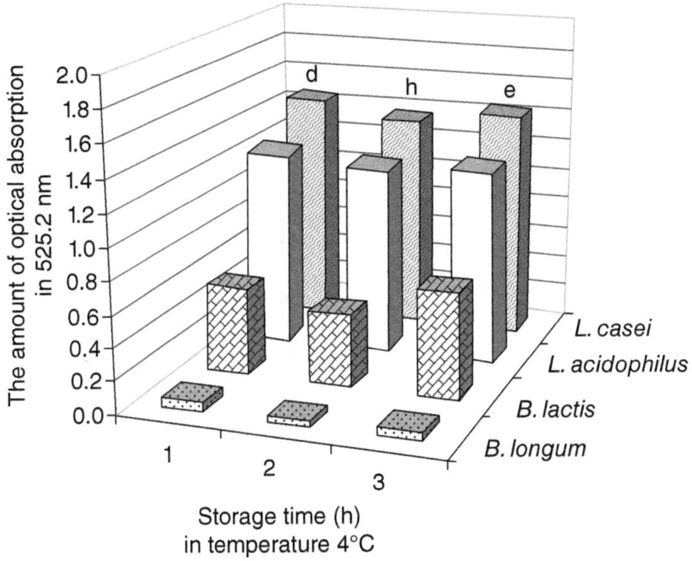

Figure 3.11 The effect of storage time (hours) at 4°C on the viability index of four probiotic bacteria.

and thus determine the best temperature, bacteria, and time separately. In these cases, the combined treatment is compared to identify the best combination of temperature × bacteria × time. The best combination of temperature × bacteria was *Lactobacillus casei* at −20°C, and the best combination of bacteria × time was *Lactobacillus casei* at one hour. The best combination of temperature × time was −20°C for three hours, and the best combination of temperature × bacteria × time was *Lactobacillus casei* at −20°C and one hour (Figures 3.11 and 3.12).

Comparisons of means in this regard, using the Duncan method at a one percent significance level, showed that the highest resistance was related to *Lactobacillus casei* at 4°C. As shown in Table 3.9, there is a significant difference between the two temperature levels at a one percent significance level. In other words, different temperatures had different effects on the viability of the bacteria. Comparisons of means in this regard, using the Duncan method at a one percent significance level, showed that the highest viability was related to 4°C for *Lactobacillus casei*. Additionally, there is a significant difference between different time levels (1, 2, and 3 months) at a one percent significance level. Comparisons of means in this regard, using the Duncan method at a one percent significance level, showed that the highest resistance was related to the first month for

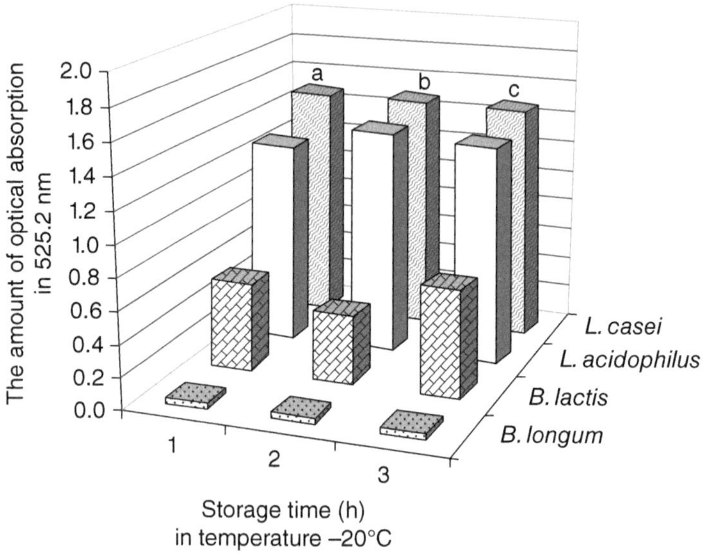

Figure 3.12 The effect of storage time (hours) at −20°C on the viability index of four probiotic bacteria.

Bifidobacterium lactis. Furthermore, there is a significant interaction effect between temperature × bacteria, bacteria × time, and temperature × time at a one percent significance level. Therefore, it is not possible to compare the average levels between different temperature levels, bacteria, and times, and thus determine the best temperature, bacteria, and time separately. In these cases, the combined treatment is compared to identify the best combination of temperature × bacteria × time. The best combination of temperature × bacteria was Lactobacillus casei at 4 and −20°C, and the best combination of bacteria × time was *Bifidobacterium lactis* in the first month. The best combination of temperature × time was 4°C for one month, and the best combination of temperature × bacteria × time was *Lactobacillus casei* at 4°C and in the first month (Figures 3.13 and 3.14).

As observed in Figures 3.13 and 3.14, among the four tested probiotic species, *Lactobacillus casei* and *Bifidobacterium lactis* exhibited good resistance to cold temperatures and showed good viability over three months of storage at 4 and −20°C. These results to some extent confirm the findings of previous studies. It has been reported that the resistance of bifidobacteria to low temperatures is lower compared to Lactobacilli. However, *Bifidobacterium lactis* was able to demonstrate good viability under these conditions. In previous studies, the effect of low storage temperatures on the viability of some probiotic species over several weeks or months has been investigated

Table 3.9 Comparisons of mean viability index of four probiotic bacteria at different temperatures over a three-month period using spectrophotometry at a wavelength of 525.2 nm with Duncan test at a 5% significance level.

Temperature (°C)	Time (month)	Bacteria	Mean viability
4	1	*Lactobacillus acidophilus*	0.0543 hd[a)]
		Bifidobacterium lactis	1.0013 d
		Lactobacillus casei	1.3793 a
		Bifidobacterium longum	0.0123 i
	2	*Lactobacillus acidophilus*	0.0527 hi
		Bifidobacterium lactis	0.8167 e
		Lactobacillus casei	1.0597 cd
		Bifidobacterium longum	0.0403 hi
	3	*Lactobacillus acidophilus*	0.0613 hi
		Bifidobacterium lactis	0.7293 f
		Lactobacillus casei	1.0597 cd
		Bifidobacterium longum	0.0403 hi
−20	1	*Lactobacillus acidophilus*	0.1057 h
		Bifidobacterium lactis	0.6973 f
		Lactobacillus casei	1.1547 b
		Bifidobacterium longum	0.0113 i
	2	*Lactobacillus acidophilus*	0.008 i
		Bifidobacterium lactis	0.4427 g
		Lactobacillus casei	1.105 bc
		Bifidobacterium longum	0 i
	3	*Lactobacillus acidophilus*	0.029 hi
		Bifidobacterium lactis	0.005 i
		Lactobacillus casei	1.1713 b
		Bifidobacterium longum	0 i

a) Nonmatching letters indicate a statistically significant difference.

and it was found that storage at freezing temperatures had no effect on the viability of these species. The fundamental issue in these studies is that they were all conducted in ice cream, under refrigeration, or under freezing conditions, and in these situations, temperature is not the only factor affecting the viability of probiotics, as viability is influenced by various factors. Although long-term studies at low temperatures during the shelf life of dairy products are necessary to identify suitable species, an important goal in these experiments was to find a rapid method for selecting probiotic

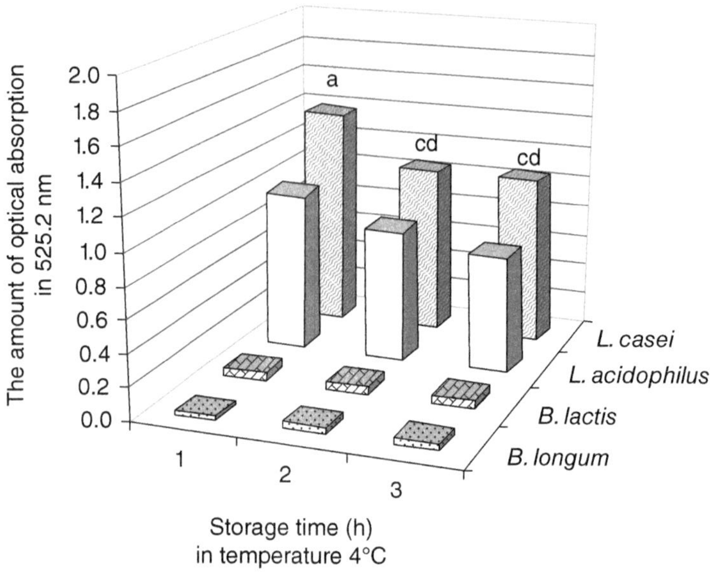

Figure 3.13 The effect of storage time (months) at 4°C on the viability index of four probiotic bacteria.

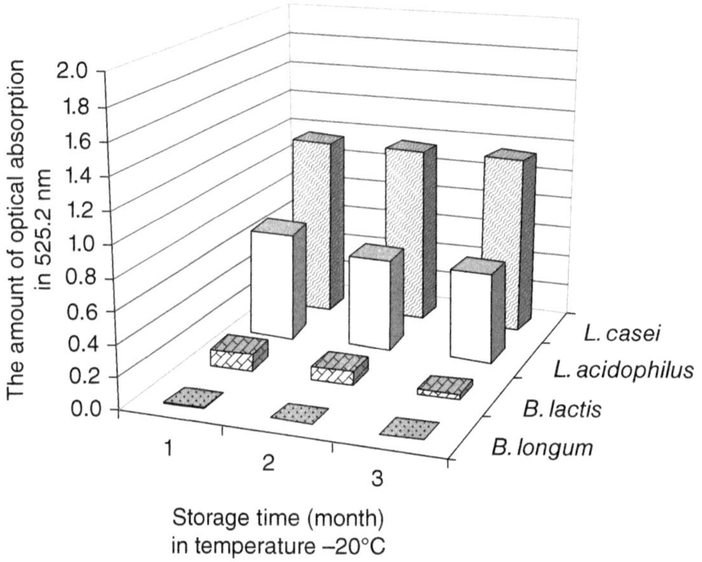

Figure 3.14 The effect of storage time (months) at −20°C on the viability index of four probiotic bacteria.

species that are resistant to low temperatures without the interference of various factors. Therefore, in this research, probiotics were cultured in MRS broth without the interference of various factors.

3.6 Selecting Resilient Probiotic Species for Use in Ice Cream

The results obtained from the treatments for each of the probiotic species were analyzed using statistical software and were compared. The species that exhibited an appropriate response to the treatment combinations and had a high growth rate and viability were selected for encapsulation and use in ice cream. The results indicated that *Lactobacillus casei* and *Bifidobacterium lactis* both had a high growth rate and demonstrated good resistance to the simulated digestive system and conditions similar to those found in ice cream, making them suitable choices for incorporation into ice cream.

3.7 Review of Researches on the Production of Functional Ice Cream

Recent two decades of research on ice cream have shown that this product possesses great potential for the distribution of *Lactobacillus acidophilus* and *Bifidobacterium bifidum* among consumers. The low storage temperature of frozen dairy products creates ideal conditions for long-term viability of bacteria. Ice cream provides a favorable environment for the high growth rate of probiotics and their survival during storage. Low-fat ice cream compared to full-fat ice cream provides better conditions for the viability of probiotic bacteria like *Lactobacillus acidophilus*, *Lactobacillus paracasei*, and *Bifidobacterium lactis*. Desserts made from milk, like frozen yoghurt, have a lower pH (around 4.5 or less), which reduces the viability of live *Lactobacillus acidophilus* and *Bifidobacterium* species. However, inoculation of probiotic bacteria into ice cream does not pose a challenge since ice cream mix has a higher pH (around 6.5–6.6), which is ideal for the survival of probiotics. Over an 11-week period of storage in low-fat fermented ice cream and frozen yoghurt, there were no significant changes observed in the initial bacterial counts. Similarly, there were no significant changes in the protein, lactose content, and sensory properties of frozen yoghurt during the storage period. Studies on the viability of *Lactobacillus johnsonii* in ice cream with varying sugar and fat levels at different temperatures showed that the count of this bacterium did not decrease during eight months of storage in the refrigerator. The count of *Lactobacillus rhamnosus* GG in ice cream with different sugar (15 and 22%) and fat (5 and 10%) levels at different temperatures (−16 and −28°C) remained unchanged over a year of storage. After six months of storage at −20°C, there was no significant change in the count of human-origin probiotic bacteria (*Lactobacillus acidophilus*, *Lactobacillus agilis*, and *Lactobacillus rhamnosus*) in ice cream containing sucrose and aspartame. *Bifidobacterium longum* and *Bifidobacterium lactis* in yoghurt fermented with vitamin C-enriched yoghurt starter culture showed no significant changes during 15 weeks of storage at −18°C. In ice cream with 4% fat content, 86–90% of *Lactobacillus acidophilus* and *Bifidobacterium animalis subsp. lactis* remained viable during two months of storage at −25°C. Inulin was found to enhance the viability of *Lactobacillus acidophilus* and *Bifidobacterium lactis* in probiotic ice cream. In sensory evaluations, fermented ice cream made with yoghurt starter and probiotics scored lower in taste and flavor compared to nonfermented ice cream (Homayouni 2008).

3.8 Investigating the Effects of Microencapsulation on the Viability of Probiotics in Various Food Products, Including Ice Cream

Microencapsulation's impact on the viability of probiotics in various food products, such as ice cream, is a recent topic that has attracted researchers' attention in the past decade. The addition of microencapsulated *Lactobacillus acidophilus* and *Bifidobacterium* species to yoghurt results in a 1–0.5 logarithmic increase in the viability of these bacteria. Two-stage microencapsulation using alginate and poly-L-lysine enhances the viability of bifidobacteria against acidic and cold (4°C) conditions. The use of 10% (w/w) of gelatin, gum arabic, and starch as encapsulating agents increases the viability of *Bifidobacterium* species during spray drying. Additionally, microencapsulation of *Bifidobacterium longum* via the spray-drying method while using whey proteins as carriers demonstrates the highest viability. Microencapsulation boosts the viability of *Bifidobacterium longum* throughout the refrigerated storage period of milk (2% fat content) compared to free cells. However, it does not protect *Bifidobacterium lactis*, *Bifidobacterium longum*, *Bifidobacterium adolescentis*, and *Bifidobacterium breve* against acidic (pH 2 and 3) and alkaline (5 and 10 g/L bile salts) conditions. Incorporating microencapsulated *Lactobacillus acidophilus* and

Bifidobacterium lactis into ice cream does not affect their viability over a six-month storage at −20°C. Alginate microencapsulation of *Lactobacillus acidophilus* and *Bifidobacterium lactis* improves their viability in cultured media and yoghurt against environmental oxygen. Microencapsulation of *Bifidobacterium breve* via spray drying with caseinates increases its viability in yoghurt during 28 days of storage at 4°C, but has no effect on *Bifidobacterium longum*. Dual-layer alginate and chitosan microencapsulation of *Lactobacillus acidophilus* and *Lactobacillus casei* effectively protects them against acidic (pH 1.5) and subsequent alkaline (0.6% bile salts) conditions, but cannot guarantee *Bifidobacterium bifidum* viability in acidic conditions. Applying post-fermented milk as a coating material in microencapsulation improves the viability of *Bifidobacterium* species during spray drying. Increasing alginate concentration from 2 to 4% enhances the viability of *Lactobacillus casei* against acidic (pH 1.5), alkaline (1 and 2% bile salts), and high-temperature (55, 60, and 65°C) conditions. Microencapsulation of *Lactobacillus acidophilus* and *Bifidobacterium lactis* in a dual-layer alginate and chitosan matrix effectively preserves their viability against adverse conditions. Incorporating microencapsulated *Lactobacillus acidophilus* and *Bifidobacterium lactis* into yoghurt increases their viability by 2 and 1 logarithmic cycles compared to free cells. This enhancement does not affect the color, flavor, or texture of yoghurt and delays secondary acidification during storage. Microencapsulation of *Lactobacillus rhamnosus* and *Bifidobacterium longum* in fermented sausages increases their viability but reduces their inhibitory effect against *Escherichia coli*. Microencapsulation of *Lactobacillus casei* and *Bifidobacterium lactis* in a calcium alginate and resistant starch matrix increases their viability by 2 logarithmic cycles in functional ice cream over six months of storage. In conclusion, microencapsulation is a suitable method for maintaining the viability of probiotic microbial cells during food production processes and facilitating their delivery of viable bacteria intestines (Homayouni et al. 2008). The future success of functional probiotic dairy foods in the market hinges on consumer acceptance of these products. The development of probiotic dairy products is a significant research priority in the field of food design and presents challenges for both the industry and the scientific community. Among functional foods, dairy probiotic products, particularly ice cream and cheese, serve as excellent vehicles for delivering probiotics to the human intestinal tract. Another strategy to maintain probiotic cell populations in the gut is by introducing prebiotics into the digestive system through regular consumption of foods containing these components. Prebiotics can create a favorable environment for the growth and activity of beneficial probiotic bacteria. Further research is essential to delve into several key areas related to probiotic dairy products:

1. **Probiotic Survival in Harsh Conditions:** More studies are needed to investigate the survival of probiotic bacteria in the challenging conditions of ice cream formulation and manufacturing. These conditions include high osmotic pressure, varying oxygen levels due to overrun, properties of packaging materials, freezing, and storage temperatures.
2. **Effects on Gut Environment:** Understanding how probiotics fare in the acidic and alkaline conditions of the human intestinal tract is crucial. This knowledge helps ensure that probiotics can reach their intended destination in the gut and provide their health benefits.
3. **Therapeutic Effects:** Assessing the therapeutic effects of live probiotic cells on human health is a critical area of investigation. This includes understanding the specific health benefits associated with different probiotic strains and their potential applications in various health conditions.

In summary, the continued development and success of probiotic dairy products, including ice cream and cheese, depend on ongoing research to optimize their formulation, ensure probiotic survival, and demonstrate their potential health benefits. These efforts aim to meet consumer expectations and contribute to improved well-being through functional dairy foods.

References

Homayouni, A. (2008). Effect of microencapsulation and resistant starch on the probiotic survival and sensory properties of synbiotic ice cream. PhD thesis. University of Tehran, Iran.

Homayouni, A., Azizi, A., Ehsani, M.R., and Yarmand, M.S. (2008). Effect of microencapsulation and resistant starch on the probiotic survival and sensory properties of synbiotic ice cream. *Food Chemistry* 111 (1): 50–55.

4

Physical Protection of Probiotics in Ice Cream Conditions

4.1 Encapsulation of Probiotic Bacteria for Use in Ice Cream

The size of the particles obtained from different methods of microencapsulation varies. In the emulsification method, particles with a diameter of 0.5–1 millimeters are produced. Using a centrifugal spray dryer, particles with an average diameter of 367 micrometers can be produced. Additionally, the spray drying method can yield particles with a diameter of 20–10 micrometers. It is noted that the size of the particles obtained from microencapsulation depends on factors such as the viscosity of the polymer solution used as the particle shell, the nozzle diameter, and the distance between the nozzle and the solidifying medium. Increasing the concentration of alginate from 1 to 4% results in larger particle size. A greater distance between the nozzle and the solidifying medium allows for the collision and fusion of particles before solidification. However, one significant consideration is that larger particles, over one millimeter in size, can cause textural roughness in the final food product and affect sensory perception. Given this, the question arises: Is there a simple method to produce smaller particles? In other words, how can the size of particles obtained through emulsification be reduced? To find answers to these questions, it is necessary to examine the factors affecting particle size in emulsification-based microencapsulation. Some of the most important factors include the rotational speed of the impeller used to disperse the core particles (bacterial cells) and the shell materials (sodium alginate and starch), the volume of the cross-linking solution (calcium chloride solution), and the volume of the oil phase. It is evident that increasing the impeller rotational speed results in smaller particle size, with particle size remaining constant when the speed reaches 400 revolutions per minute. When a single-blade impeller

Probiotic Ice Cream: Science and Technology, First Edition. Aziz Homayouni-Rad.

rotates at a speed of 400 revolutions per minute, particles with the minimum diameter are formed. Consequently, in the subsequent stages, a speed of 400 revolutions per minute was selected as the basis for producing particles with a diameter under 100 micrometers. Initially, the alginate/starch/bacterial mixture was added drop by drop to the oil using a pipette to create a uniform emulsion with a smaller particle size while stirring the mixture. However, since the alginate/starch/bacterial mixture needed to ultimately form an emulsion, adding the mixture to the oil all at once made no difference. Therefore, in all experiments, the alginate/starch/bacterial mixture was added to the oil as a whole. To ensure the sterility of the resulting particles, the alginate solution was sterilized in an autoclave (121°C for 15 minutes). However, several attempts at microencapsulation using sterile sodium alginate solution did not yield satisfactory results, and the particles did not form. It was assumed that the lack of particle formation was likely due to the heating of the sodium alginate solution. Therefore, in the subsequent stages, all glassware and materials used, except for the alginate, were sterilized. Weighing and transferring alginate to the solution under sterile conditions were performed to obtain sterile particles. When the alginate solution is heated, the polymer loses its ability to form a soft gel, preventing the formation of particles. It has been shown that 2% cornstarch (resistant starch) plays a role in the viability of probiotics. Resistant starch is considered a prebiotic compound that reaches the large intestine for probiotic consumption. Amylose-resistant starch enhances the survival of *Bifidobacteria* under acidic and alkaline conditions in the digestive system. Therefore, the use of 2% cornstarch is believed to enhance the survival of probiotics in dairy products and the human digestive system. Additionally, the use of 2% cornstarch increases the microencapsulation efficiency. Adding 30% glycerol along with 2% alginate and 2% cornstarch can prevent the reduction in the number of viable probiotic cells during freezing of the cells along with the culture medium at −20°C. In fact, glycerol and resistant starch act as protective compounds against freezing. Research has shown that sucrose, polydextrose, and dextrin have a protective effect on the survival of *Lactobacillus rhamnosus* during freeze-drying. Synbiotic ice cream was created using traditional ice cream production techniques, which included 1% resistant starch as a prebiotic ingredient and two strains of lactic acid bacteria (*Lactobacillus casei* and *Bifidobacterium lactis*) as probiotic bacteria. The viability of both microencapsulated and free probiotics within the ice cream was assessed over a six-month storage period at −20°C. It was found that microencapsulated probiotics within alginate-starch beads exhibited a 30% higher survival rate compared to nonencapsulated bacteria. Consequently, the number of viable probiotic bacteria in the functional ice cream exceeded 10^9 CFU/g within two months, surpassing the recommendation of the International Dairy Federation (10^7 CFU/g). In conclusion, synbiotic ice cream represents an effective vehicle for delivering probiotics in the human diet (Homayouni et al. 2008).

4.2 Encapsulation

Microencapsulation, also known as encapsulation, is a process through which a thin and continuous coating is formed around various substances (solid particles, liquid droplets, and gas bubbles). The capsule wall (shell) encloses the encapsulated materials. In other words, microencapsulation is the technology of packaging fine solid, liquid, and gas particles inside very small capsules, which release their contents under specific conditions of shear stress, temperature, enzymes, pH, fermentation, etc., after a certain period of time. The difference between this process and trapping is the possibility of capturing a certain amount of trapped compound on the surface of the trap particles. In trapping, the desired compounds are trapped inside or throughout the gel or crystal matrix. The materials inside the capsules in the microencapsulation process are referred to as active materials, inner phases, core materials, or payloads. The materials that provide the coating are known as shell, cover, wall materials, carriers, or encapsulants. The thickness and number of coating layers can vary. Figure 4.1 illustrates the types of capsules obtained from microencapsulation. Microencapsulation, also referred to as microencapsulating or microcoating, is a term used to describe coating particles with a diameter of 0.2–5000 micrometers. Particles larger than 5000 micrometers (5 millimeters) are classified as macrocapsules, and particles smaller than 0.2 micrometers fall into the category of nanomicrocapsules. When the encapsulated materials are very large, the process is called coating or covering. Generally, microencapsulated particles are spherical in shape, although the structure of the materials inside the capsules can influence the final shape of the particles. Encapsulated food ingredients may include enzymes, flavorings, taste enhancers, sweeteners, antioxidants, food preservatives, acidulants, amino acids, colorants, oil particles, fats, emulsifiers, vitamins, salts, and microorganisms like lactic acid bacteria. The microencapsulation process is not only used in the food industry but also in various other industries such as pharmaceuticals, biotechnology, and the chemical industry. It has been shown that microencapsulation can act as a barrier to protect microencapsulated cells from moisture, oxygen, and acids. It also provides good protection against high temperature and pressure for a short period of time (Homayouni 2008).

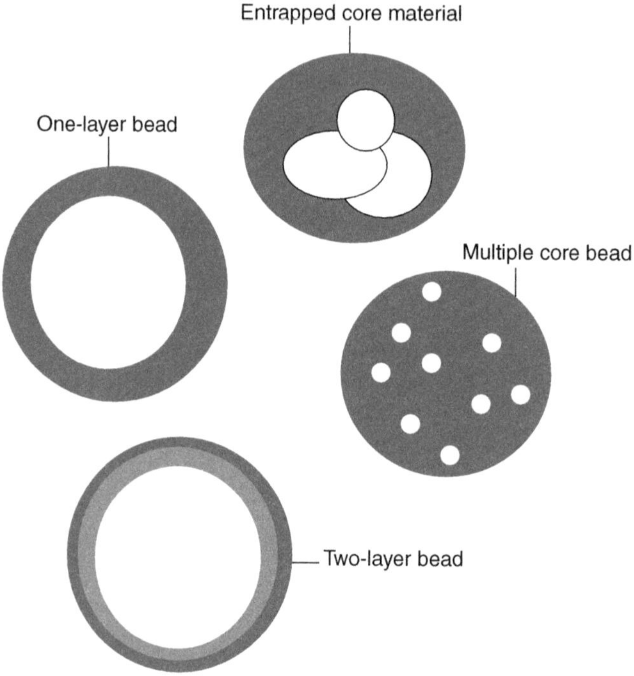

Figure 4.1 Types of capsules obtained from microencapsulation.

4.2.1 Applications of Microencapsulation

In 1954 AD, microencapsulation was first used to create carbonless copy paper. In this process, colorless dye precursors are microencapsulated at sizes of about 20 micrometers and sprayed as a very thin layer onto the back of the top paper. The bottom paper is coated with a layer of colorless developer. When something is written on the top paper, the pressure from the pen tip breaks the capsules, releasing the colorless dye precursor. This precursor reacts with the developer on the bottom paper upon contact, forming a colored image. Microencapsulation finds numerous applications in the food industry. It is used to stabilize encapsulated materials, control the onset of reactions, regulate the time and rate of material release, mask flavors, colors, and odors, detect pressures, enhance shelf life, protect food compounds, preserve nutritional value, transform liquids into solids, reduce volatilization, and keep active ingredients separate. For instance, the shelf life of raw milk can be extended by adding calcium alginate microcapsules containing lactic acid bacteria such as *Lactococcus lactis* and *Lactobacillus helveticus*. Similarly, the shelf life of dairy products made from raw milk can also be increased using this method. These specific bacteria reduce the activity of spoilage bacteria in milk by up to 50%. Furthermore, the immobilization of fermentation cells can decrease fermentation time and make the cells reusable. Liquid culture bacteria need to remain alive to be beneficial to their host. Hence, they not only need to survive the passage through the digestive system but also during food storage. Microencapsulation can protect food components against factors like processing temperature, humidity, and other food components. Probiotic bacteria, for example, require protection during their passage through the gastrointestinal tract to ensure their viability. Bifidobacteria can be inoculated into cheese by microencapsulation with calcium alginate capsules. One reason for microencapsulation of food components is to delay their release during processing. For example, artificial sweeteners can be encapsulated and released under high cooking temperatures to maintain their sweetness. Controlled release of probiotics within food is achieved through mechanisms such as:

1. Pressure-induced release: applying pressure to the capsule wall causes the encapsulated material to exit.
2. Diffusion-induced release: encapsulated material diffuses through the polymer capsule wall or pores in the wall.
3. Osmotic release: high osmotic pressure within the capsule forces the material to be released.
4. Membrane changes: removing a control portion of the capsule wall triggers the material to be released.
5. Solvent-induced release: swelling of the capsule wall upon contact with a solvent releases the material.
6. Enzyme-induced release: specific enzymes trigger the release of encapsulated materials.
7. Temperature-induced release: changes in temperature cause the material inside the capsule to be released.
8. Wall melting: heat melts the capsule wall, releasing the encapsulated material.
9. Combination mechanisms: a combination of the above mechanisms causes the material inside the capsule to be released.

The actual mechanism of material release from within the capsules can be achieved through one of the above-mentioned methods or a combination of them. These mechanisms depend on the type of capsule wall material, the intended application, and the nature of the encapsulated materials. The capsule wall material needs to form a thin, film-like layer around the core materials quickly and should not react with the encapsulated materials. Additionally, the capsule wall and core materials should not mix with each other. On the other hand, capsule wall materials must be resistant during storage, transportation, and transfer in the environment they are used. At times, alginate capsules containing lactic acid bacteria are coated with a layer of poly-L-lysine to minimize the release of cells. This additional coating can enhance the resistance of the capsule to external factors and promote controlled release (Homayouni 2009).

4.2.2 Materials Used in Microencapsulation

In general, the hydrocolloids used in microencapsulation should form a suitable and stable emulsion, exhibit good retention properties for the core materials during processing and storage, and allow for a proper release of these materials. The carriers (encapsulants) used for cell immobilization can be categorized into two types: organic and inorganic. Organic carriers include polysaccharides, proteins, and synthetic polymers. Polysaccharide carriers encompass agar, agarose, alginate, carrageenan, cellulose, dextran, pectin, and lignin from wood. Proteins such as collagen, egg white, and gelatin are used as proteinaceous carriers. Synthetic polymers include polyacrylamide, phenolic resins, polystyrene, and polyurethane. Inorganic carriers consist of fats, emulsifiers, small-molecule sugars, and polymers. The choice of materials for microencapsulation depends on the physical and chemical properties of the core materials and the encapsulation method. These materials should be nonsoluble and nonreactive with the core materials. Substances such as gums, gelatin, agar, alginate, modified alginate with polyethylene imine, carrageenan, chitosan, gum arabic, and phosphorylated starches are utilized in the construction of microcapsules. The stability of ionotropic gels such as alginate, carrageenan, chitosan, agar, and gum arabic in the capsule wall depends on the ionic conditions in the surrounding medium. These materials are often used for immobilization of microbial cells. The advantage of using natural polymers for microorganism microencapsulation lies in their nontoxicity and compatibility with the microbes. For instance, bifidobacteria remain more viable in alginate beads than in carrageenan beads. Various factors such as molecular weight, solubility, film formation, permeability, crystallization, and glass transition play a role in the selection of encapsulant materials. At low temperatures and water activities, polymeric materials are in a glassy state and restrict molecular diffusion. At higher temperatures and water activities, encapsulant materials become elastic and allow increased molecular diffusion. This property allows encapsulant materials to regulate the release and diffusion processes of the encapsulated core materials. Moreover, in the food industry, the effects of encapsulant materials on taste, texture, and cost are also considered. It has been shown that microcapsules made from pectin and casein have the ability to maintain the viability of probiotics during the drying process of microcapsules and also in simulated digestion conditions.

4.2.2.1 Calcium Alginate

Mostly, sodium alginate along with multivalent ions is used for cell immobilization. In this method, cells are mixed with a sodium alginate solution, and then droplets of this mixture are added to a solution of calcium chloride. The advantage of this method lies in its ability to maintain the viability of microbial cells. However, when using destabilizing agents like phosphate buffers or citrates, cell destruction might occur. The strength and porosity of microcapsules can be controlled by choosing an appropriate concentration of alginate. The tighter the gel structure will be when there is a higher proportion of L-gluronic acid in the alginate structure. Furthermore, increasing the proportion of D-mannuronic acid leads to larger openings between alginate microcapsules. With increasing alginate concentration, the mechanical strength of the microcapsules increases, but as the cellular mass increases, the strength of microcapsules decreases. The diffusion coefficient of glucose and ethanol through alginate membranes decreases with higher alginate concentrations. The conditions of operation are crucial for immobilizing Chlorella cells in alginate, particularly when aiming for greater microcapsule stability. Trivalent ions are advantageous for enhancing the strength of calcium alginate microcapsules. Calcium alginate gel and pre-made cellulose microcapsules are used for immobilizing *Lactobacillus acidophilus* cells. Temperature and drying conditions do not significantly affect the number of immobilized cells. Cellular immobilization leads to an increase in acetic acid production. When *Saccharomyces cerevisiae* cells are encapsulated in spherical and cylindrical alginate matrices at low density, individual colonies form within the gel network due to cellular growth. In alginate microcapsules, these colonies are stretched and form lentil-shaped structures with their longitudinal axes oriented along the surface of the microcapsules. Conversely, cylindrical-shaped microcapsules yield colonies that are spherical and nonuniformly distributed, with no particular arrangement in terms of length and width. The average diameter of pores and gaps in calcium alginate gel at concentrations of 0.5 and 3% is 17 and 14.7 nm, respectively. The mechanical strength of calcium alginate gel decreases in the presence of microbial cells due to the inhibition of hydrogen bonding. The mechanical strength of calcium alginate and barium alginate gels gradually decreases during storage, reaching the initial level after 30 days and decreasing further until 90 days after gel preparation. The stability of calcium alginate gels cross-linked with calcium bridges

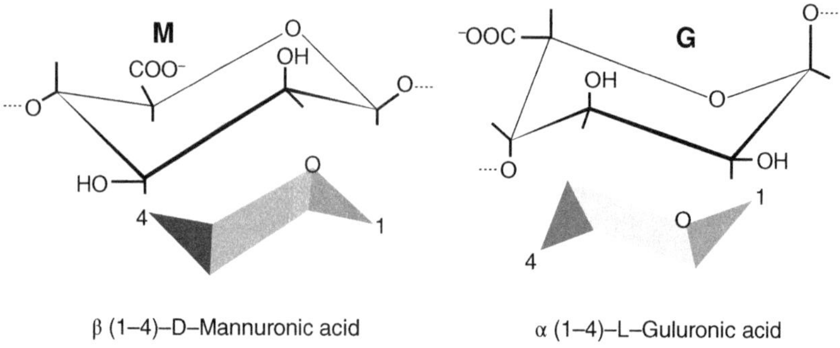

Figure 4.2 Chemical structure of alginate.

decreases over 60 days after preparation, with a focus on protein molecule diffusion with molecular weights ranging from 14.5 to 155 kDa. Studies indicate an increase in the average diameter of pores and gaps in calcium alginate gel over 60 days, from 6.17 to 9.28 nm. Alginate is employed for immobilizing bacterial, algal, fungal, plant, and animal cells. The chemical structure of alginate is shown in Figure 4.2. While various materials are available for microcapsule shell formation, calcium alginate is frequently used for microencapsulation of microbial cells, particularly lactic acid bacteria. Figure 4.3 illustrates a microscopic image of microencapsulated probiotic bacteria in a mixture of alginate and starch. Calcium alginate is nontoxic and is used as a food additive and carrier for pharmaceutical agents. The advantages of using alginate over other materials include its cost-effectiveness, ease of application, rapid gel formation with divalent ions like calcium, heat stability, reversible gelation, and long-term viability preservation of microorganisms (Homayouni 2009).

Alginate-based microcapsules, due to their gel structure being dependent on ion reactions, can easily undergo reversible changes. This means that by substituting with cation-exchange materials such as phosphates and altering the concentration and pH of the solution, the gel structure of alginate can be disrupted, and the encapsulating shell can break. Alginate is a natural polymer derived from brown algae, in which units of beta-D-mannuronic acid and alpha-L-gluronic acid are connected by glycoside bonds (1→4) (Figure 4.4). Cells encapsulated with alginate often have an extended viability period after freeze-drying. The diffusion coefficients of ethanol and glucose in calcium alginate are only about 9% less than that in water, making them nearly equivalent to water diffusion. Conversely, the diffusion coefficient (permeability) of oxygen in barium alginate is only 25% of that in water. These features allow microencapsulated cells to remain

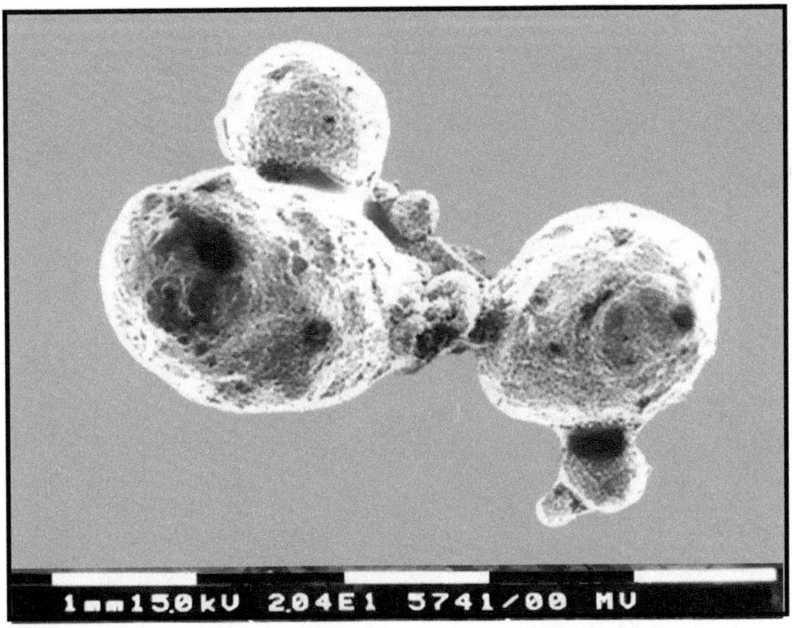

Figure 4.3 Microscopic image of microencapsulated probiotic bacteria in a mixture of alginate and starch (droplet size of the capsules is approximately 1–2 millimeters).

viable within the capsules while restricting their rapid growth. Limited growth inside the capsules is essential to prevent enzyme inactivation. However, excessive growth can lead to leakage of cellular contents, capsule rupture, accumulation of toxic by-products, and decreased production efficiency (Homayouni 2009).

4.2.2.2 Resistant Starch

Resistant starch refers to certain types of starch products that are not absorbed in the small intestine of adults and are therefore considered prebiotic compounds. These substances reach the large intestine for consumption by probiotics. The consumption of resistant starch in the large intestine by probiotics leads to the production of beneficial cellular metabolites, such as short-chain fatty acids, and prevents intestinal diseases. Resistant starch, in addition to its therapeutic effects, improves the appearance, texture, and mouth feel of food compared to regular dietary fibers. There are four types of resistant starch:

1. The first type is starch trapped within seed cells, such as legumes.
2. The second type is natural starch granules found in bananas and potatoes.

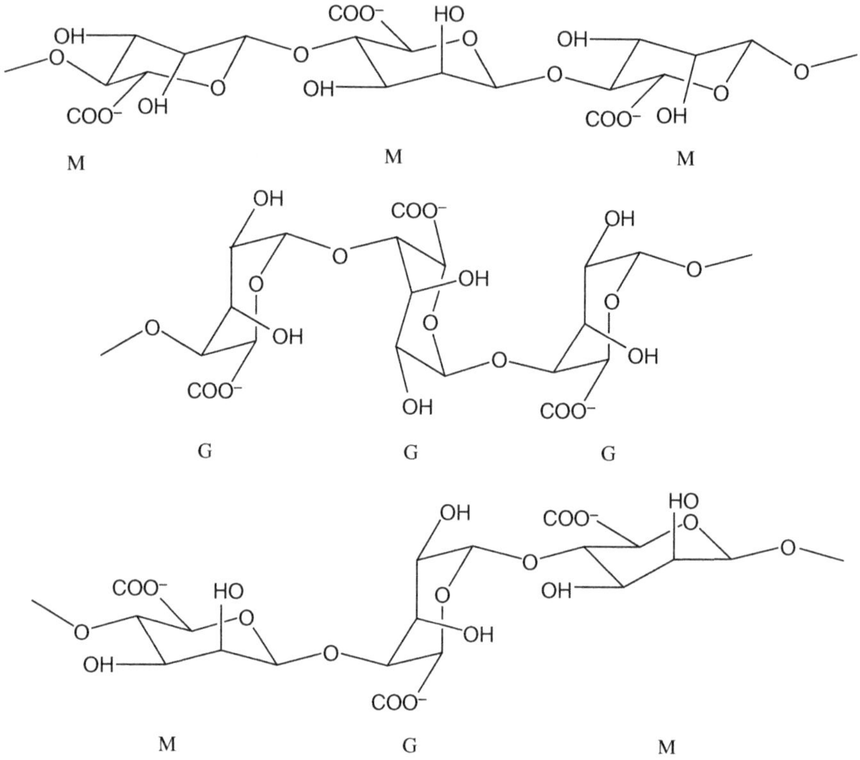

Figure 4.4 Chemical structure of the constitutive units of alginate: Mannuronic acid (M) and Gluronic acid (G).

3. The third type includes products resulting from retrograded starch in bread and boiled potatoes.
4. The fourth type is modified starch due to Maillard reactions, caramelization, esterification, and etherification, which forms new glycoside bonds and inhibits the action of alpha-amylase enzymes on starch.

Starch is found in two forms in nature: amylose and amylopectin. Only amylose is classified as resistant starch and is involved in the phenomenon of retrogradation. The formation of resistant starch depends on various factors, including temperature, water content, and fat. Only 20% of resistant starch is produced from corn starch during autoclaving. By subjecting it to high-pressure heat and subsequent cooling up to 20 times, the production yield of resistant starch can be increased by 40%. The optimal amylose-to-water ratio for resistant starch production is

Table 4.1 Resistant starch content in common foods.

Food type	Resistant starch to total starch ratio (%)
Bread	2.2–4.3
Breakfast cereals	0–9
Whole grain cereals	1.7–12.3
Potato	0.6–9
Pasta	1.3–4.2

1 to 3.5 (weight-to-weight). Fats form complexes with amylose, preventing the formation of resistant starch. Type 3-resistant starch comprises 60–70% double-helix polyglucan segments with alpha-(1→4) linkage and only 25–30% crystalline structure. The presence of a high amount of double-helix segments (similar to beta-type amylose) appears to limit the activity of alpha-amylase. As shown in Table 4.1, resistant starch accounts for less than 5% of the dry matter in processed foods (Homayouni 2009).

Resistant amylose starch, considered a type of resistant starch, enhances the survival of bifidobacteria against the conditions of the digestive system. Therefore, it has been claimed that the use of 2% corn starch (amylose) is capable of increasing the viability of probiotics in both food products and the human digestive system. Additionally, the application of 2% corn starch increases encapsulation efficiency. The use of amylose corn starch along with specific bifidobacterial strains in laboratory animal feed has shown heightened synergistic or greater synbiotic effects compared to the use of bifidobacteria with digestible (normal) starch. Furthermore, after discontinuation of probiotic consumption, if resistant starch is included in livestock feed, the probiotic population remains significantly higher for up to one week compared to normal starch (Figure 4.5). This phenomenon indicates that resistant starch reaches the consumption of utilized probiotics (bifidobacterial strains) in the large intestine. When resistant starch is consumed by humans along with the probiotic bacterium *Clostridium butyricum*, it reduces the number of markers for colorectal cancer better than when probiotics are used alone (Homayouni 2009).

4.2.3 Methods of Encapsulation

Depending on the type of encapsulating material, the nature of the coating material, and the intended applications of the resulting microcapsules,

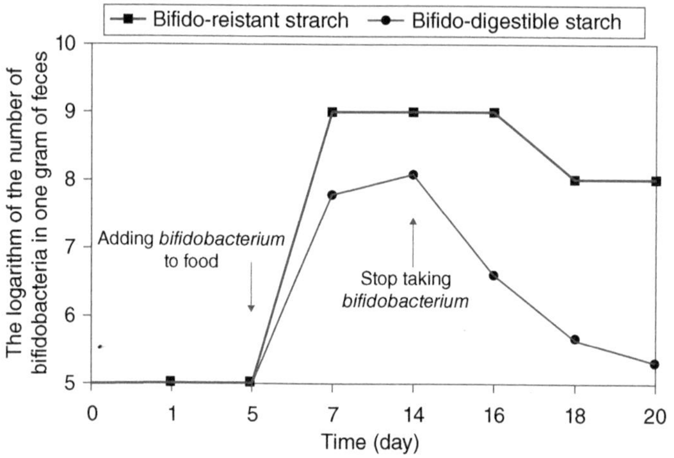

Figure 4.5 Synergistic effect of resistant starch on bifidobacteria in laboratory animals.

various methods of encapsulation have been developed. The size of microcapsules in each encapsulation method is specific. Encapsulation methods include static nozzle spraying, centrifugal nozzle spraying, phase separation of suspensions through a rotating disc, floating nozzle, oscillating nozzle, rotating disc, spray drying, fluidized bed coating, air-suspension coating, internal polymerization, electrostatic deposition, turbine coating, solvent evaporation, emulsification encapsulation, molecular coating with beta-cyclodextrin, simultaneous crystallization, and in situ polymerization. In the food industry, due to the sensitivity of core materials, the required size of microcapsules, physicochemical properties of core and shell materials, type of application for coated materials, mechanism of core release, and economic considerations, an appropriate encapsulation method can be chosen. Various industrial and semi-industrial processes have been investigated for microcapsule preparation. For instance, nozzles positioned on a continuously rotating ring have been used to spray alginate and cell suspensions into a cross-linking solution. In this method, cross-linking solution forms lateral connections between alginate molecules, resulting in the solidification of microcapsules. Another method involves using a nozzle with two intersecting conduits, through which microbial cells are ejected from the internal needle and sodium alginate from the external needle under the influence of airflow, subsequently entering a calcium chloride solution (Homayouni 2009).

4.2.3.1 Spray Drying Encapsulation

In the food industry, due to its cost-effectiveness, spray drying is commonly used for encapsulation. Advantages of this method include the stability of the formed coating, the rapid solubility of microcapsules due to their small size, and the availability of spraying equipment. However, this system also has its drawbacks. Coating materials at high concentrations can create high viscosity, and the heat used in spray drying may lead to the degradation or oxidation of active core materials and possible reactions with solvents. Moreover, this method is not suitable for foods with moderate moisture content. Spray drying is used for encapsulating sugars, polysaccharides, starch, proteins, vitamins, colorants, fats and oils, flavor compounds, and enhancers. The coating materials used in this method include carbohydrates such as dextrin or simple sugars, starch (regular and modified), and gums like Farsi gum (acacia gum), or proteins such as gelatin and soy protein, as well as cellulose esters and ethers. The process of coating food compounds using spray drying is initiated by first turning the core and coating materials into an emulsion or suspension in a solvent. This mixture is then atomized into fine particles (atomization) using a nozzle Figure 4.6. Contact between these tiny droplets and hot air inside the drying chamber causes the solvent to evaporate, resulting in the formation of a shell around the core material. Water is often the solvent used in this method. Due to its high-speed process, spray drying is highly suitable for heat-sensitive food compounds. Additionally, as depicted in Figure 4.7, spray drying might involve liquid nitrogen spraying and freeze-drying in a vacuum (Homayouni 2009).

4.2.3.2 Centrifugal Nozzle Spraying Encapsulation

In this method, core materials such as essential oils, flavor enhancers, vitamins, micronutrients, acids, colors, spices, and water-soluble solutions are in liquid form at room temperature and exhibit low viscosity. Suitable shell materials for this method include gelatin, sodium alginate, carrageenan, starch, cellulose derivatives, Farsi gum, fats and fatty acids, wax, polyethylene glycol, or mixtures of these compounds. This process requires a rotary centrifugal nozzle device, where liquid core materials are pumped from the inner tube and shell materials from the outer tube. Consequently, at the nozzle outlet, a column of shell materials forms around the core materials. With the rotation of the device, the column of materials breaks into fine droplets and forms microcapsules. The mechanism of centrifugal nozzle spraying encapsulation is depicted in Figure 4.8. As seen in Figure 4.9, centrifugal spraying technology can be employed for semi-industrial scale encapsulation of lactic acid bacteria (Homayouni 2009).

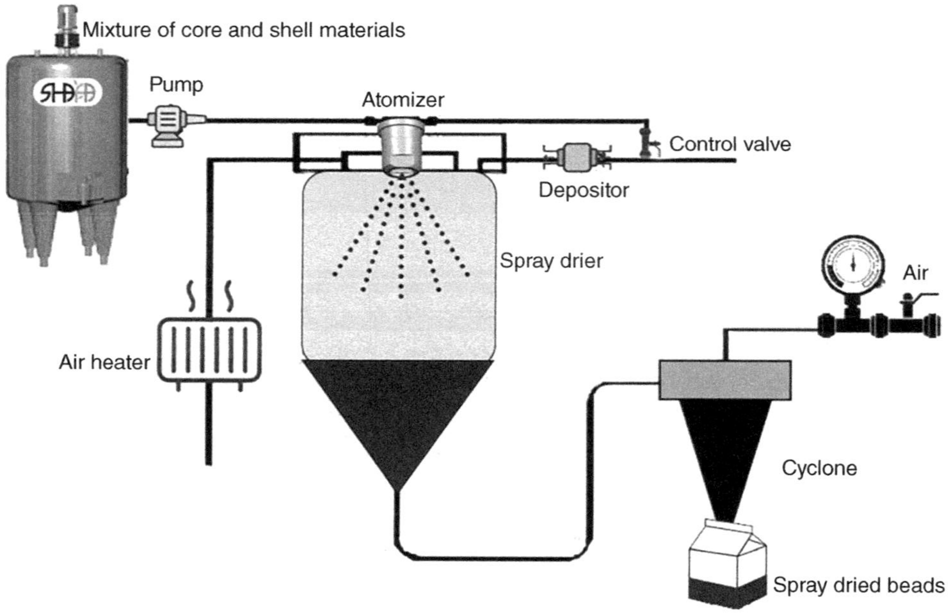

Figure 4.6 Process of spray drying encapsulation in hot air.

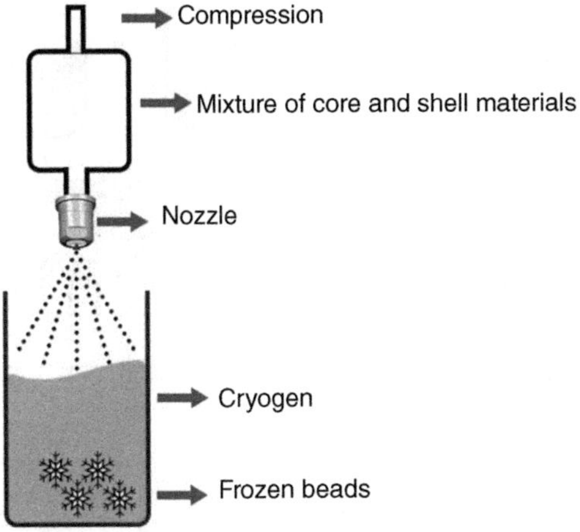

Figure 4.7 Process of spray drying encapsulation using liquid nitrogen spraying and freeze-drying.

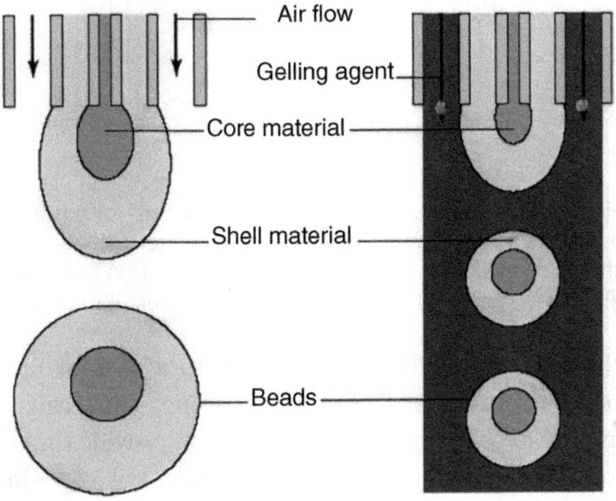

Figure 4.8 Mechanism of operation for encapsulation using the centrifugal nozzle spraying method.

4.2.3.3 Emulsification-based Encapsulation

Microencapsulation and entrapment in emulsion are frequently employed in the pharmaceutical industry and have recently become common in the food industry as well. Emulsification-based encapsulation is easily scalable. The advantage of this method lies in producing smaller microcapsules that prevent undesired changes in food texture. In this process, active core materials are added to a hydrocolloidal solution (aqueous solution). Subsequently, a significant amount of oil is added to the aqueous solution, and the resulting mixture is homogenized. Eventually, the polymer dissolved in water either precipitates or forms cross-links, creating small gels around the core materials, which float within the oil phase. In the traditional method for preparing calcium alginate microcapsules, calcium

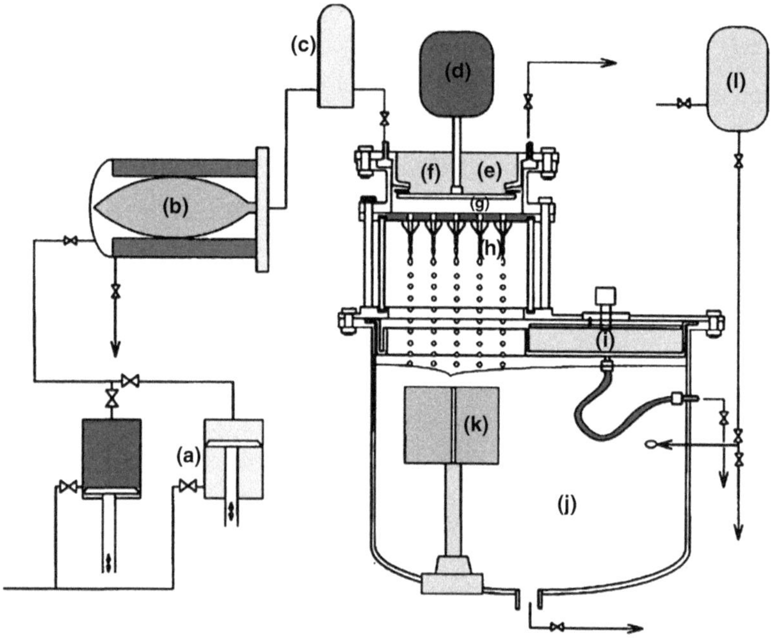

Figure 4.9 Schematic of a multinozzle system for encapsulation. (a) Dual-piston pump, (b) Sterile chamber, (c) Airflow regulator, (d) Vibrating system, (e) Pulsation chamber membrane, (f) Coaxial slits, (g) Pulsation chamber, (h) Nozzle plate, (i) Bypass system, (j) Reaction vessel, (k) Stirrer, (l) Cross-linker solution inlet.

chloride was added drop by drop to a sodium alginate solution. Later, calcium ethylene diamine tetra-acetic acid (calcium-EDTA) was used instead of calcium chloride, as it could provide the necessary calcium ions for gel formation (Figure 4.10). A mixture of 3% alginate along with starter bacteria can be dropwise added to vegetable oil containing 2.0% Tween 80 (polyoxyethylene sorbitan mono-oleate), followed by firming the resulting microcapsules with calcium chloride and separating them using centrifugation, then washing with sterile water. This method can be used to protect probiotics in dairy products. Furthermore, microcapsules can be recoated with a more resistant shell. During encapsulation, microcapsules with a single probiotic strain or a mixture of probiotic strains can be prepared. Successful encapsulation can also be achieved by applying the reverse procedure. In this approach, *L. casei* cells are mixed with sterile calcium chloride solution and then dropwise added using a syringe to a 0.6% sodium alginate solution (containing 1.0% Tween 20). Finally, the excess sodium alginate is washed off with sterile saline solution, and the microcapsules are set with a 1% calcium chloride solution (Homayouni 2009).

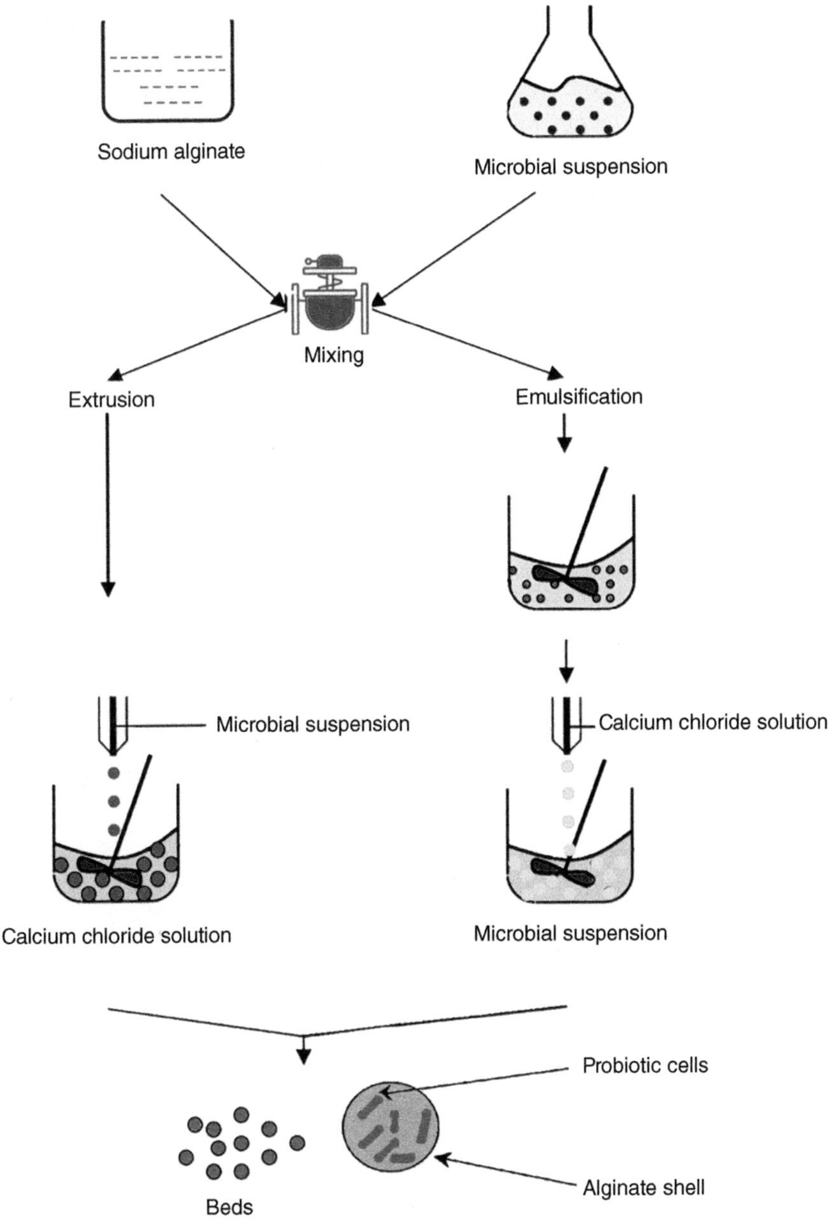

Figure 4.10 Encapsulation of bacteria using the spray drying and emulsification methods.

References

Homayouni, A. (2008). Effect of microencapsulation and resistant starch on the probiotic survival and sensory properties of synbiotic ice cream. PhD thesis. University of Tehran, Iran.

Homayouni, A. (2009). *Therapeutical effects of functional probiotic, prebiotic and synbiotic foods*. Tabriz, Iran: Published by Tabriz University of Medical Sciences.

Homayouni, A., Azizi, A., Ehsani, M.R., and Yarmand, M.S. (2008). Effect of microencapsulation and resistant starch on the probiotic survival and sensory properties of synbiotic ice cream. *Food Chemistry* 111 (1): 50–55.

5

Nutritional Value of Functional Ice Cream

5.1 Nutritional Value of Ice Cream

Ice cream, a delicious dairy food, is known for its high nutritional value and has been enjoyed as a frozen dessert for many years. Today, the ice cream industry has undergone significant development, and the technology of ice cream production, preservation, and distribution has become an advanced indicator of a country's progress. Various types of ice creams are produced worldwide, including low-fat ice cream, full-fat ice cream, regular ice cream, lactose-free ice cream, probiotic ice cream (medicinal), powdered ice cream, sorbet, and fruit-flavored ice cream, each available in different flavors, colors, and shapes. Low-fat ice cream has become common, especially in advanced societies where calorie reduction in their diet is of utmost importance, and its consumption continues to rise. On the other hand, due to lactose intolerance, which results from a lack of the lactase enzyme in the digestive system, people in many parts of the world avoid consuming dairy products containing lactose. In such cases, lactose-free ice cream can be used without causing any problems. Additionally, probiotic ice cream has medicinal properties. The microorganisms present in this type of ice cream can eliminate harmful microbes in the digestive system, aiding in improving health. As a result, the production of this type of product is crucial, particularly in developing countries. Probiotic science and technology has been an ever-growing field in recent decades. Thus, it has opened new vistas of potential research in fermented food formulation and manufacturing. This book is compiled into three sections with 12 chapters highlighting different aspects varying from selection of appropriate probiotic strains for use in ice cream to formulation and characterization of final product. It is designed fundamentally to be a reference book to the experts providing a passage for future researches. So, this book may fill up the gap between

Probiotic Ice Cream: Science and Technology, First Edition. Aziz Homayouni-Rad.

probiotic science and probiotic technology to manufacture probiotic ice cream and frozen dairy products (Homayouni, 2008).

5.1.1 Energy Content of Ice Cream

The unit commonly used by nutrition experts to measure and express the energy required by the body and the energy content of foods is kcal. Each kcal is equivalent to the amount of heat required to raise the temperature of one kilogram of water by 1°C. Digestion of a food substance involves breaking it down into simple nutrients in the digestive system for absorption. The metabolism of absorbed substances involves chemical changes from the moment of absorption until they are eliminated from the body. Metabolism includes processes such as nutrient distribution in the body, tissue repair and breakdown (anabolism and catabolism), and energy absorption and release. Nutrients need to be present in the diet in the same proportion as the body requires. As seen in Table 5.1, the energy content and nutritional components of ice cream depend on the nutritional value of the ingredients used in its preparation. Different dairy products are used in various proportions in ice cream production. The fat and protein content of ice cream is generally 3–4 and 12–16% higher, respectively, than that of milk. Additionally, ice cream may contain other food products such as fruits, nuts, eggs, pastries, and sugar, which significantly enhance its nutritional value. The solid components of milk in ice cream undergo more heat treatment compared to milk pasteurization. Furthermore, during the freezing process, ice cream mixtures tolerate very low temperatures and

Table 5.1 Composition per 100 grams of regular ice cream.

Components	Sorbet	Sherbet	For ice cream with different fat contents				Regular ice cream
			16%	12%	10%	5%	
Water (%)	66.9	8.9	62.8	62.1	63.2	66.7	61.7
Energy (kcal)	78	377	222	207	193	152	196.7
Protein (%)	0.4	10	2.6	4	4.5	4.8	4.1
Total fat (%)	Negligible	2.4	16.1	12.5	10.6	5.1	12
Weight equivalent to 100 kcal (grams)	128.4	26.5	45	48.3	51.7	65.6	50.8
Total carbohydrates (%)	32.6	26.5	18	20.6	20.8	22.4	20.7

can be stored for much longer periods before consumption. However, ice cream is not a significant source of iron or trace minerals. Ice cream serves as an energy source. Since the compounds in ice cream are almost fully absorbed by the body, it is considered suitable for the growth of children and individuals requiring weight gain. Consequently, its consumption should be controlled for those aiming to lose or maintain weight.

5.1.2 Caloric Content of Ice Cream

The caloric content of ice cream is crucial for its inclusion on labels for producers, and on the other hand, it is highly valuable for nutrition experts and dietary advisors to provide useful dietary recommendations. The caloric content of ice cream generally depends on the percentage of carbohydrates and lactose, sweeteners, many filling ingredients, sugar present in fruits, flavor and aroma enhancers, the percentage of milk protein, fat substitutes (based on whey protein), nuts, eggs, and cocoa. The caloric content of each gram of fat, protein, and carbohydrates, as measured by a calorimeter, is approximately 9.45, 5.65, and 4.10 kcal, respectively. Not all digestible food substances are absorbed by the body; on average, 5% of fats, 8% of proteins, and 2% of carbohydrates are not absorbed. Therefore, the expected caloric content of each gram of fat, protein, and carbohydrates in milk is 8.79, 4.27, and 3.87 kcal, respectively. Scientific experiences have rounded these figures to 9, 4, and 4. Minerals and vitamins do not contain significant energy content. The metabolic value of each type of carbohydrate has very little connection with the type of carbohydrate; all carbohydrates have the same energy yield. The caloric value of 100 grams of ice cream containing 12.5% fat, 11% nonfat solids, 15% sugar, and 0.3% gelatin is calculated as follows (assuming that lactose and protein in nonfat milk solids are 52 and 36%, respectively):

Fat	$12.5 \times 9 = 112.50$
Carbohydrates	$[15 \times (11 \times 0.52)] = 82.88$
Protein	$[(11 \times 0.36) + 0.30] \times 4 = 17.04$
Total	212.42

The caloric content of a serving of ice cream depends on the composition of the ice cream mixture and the weight of each gallon of the final ice cream product. The serving size used for nutritional studies for an ice cream serving is half a cup or 120 grams. For "Sweet Frozen Ice Cream," frozen flavored and aromatic products, "Pops Ice Cream," and frozen fruit extracts, the weight of a serving is considered to be 85 grams. The scale for "sundae" (ice cream containing walnut kernels) is also one cup. It is evident that the weight of an ice cream serving and its components are the major variable factors in its energy content. Ice cream is sold by volume, and its specific weight is lower. The weight of ice cream can be calculated by multiplying the mixture's density by the volume at the time of product delivery. Density is a function of the volume expansion coefficient of the product and its composition. It varies between 1.06 and 1.15 g/mL. When the volume expansion coefficient is 100%, each ice cream serving weighs 63–68 grams. If the volume expansion coefficient is 50%, the weight of the ice cream will be 94–120 grams. For example, the caloric content of an ice cream with high fat and dry matter, containing 16% fat, 10% nonfat solid milk, and 17% sweetener (by weight), and with a volume expansion coefficient of 100% after freezing, can be calculated as follows:

1. First, the density of the mixture is calculated. For this purpose, the density of fat, nonfat solids, and water is assumed to be 0.93, 1.58, and 1 g/mL, respectively.
2. The weight of a 120-gram mixture (corresponding to 118.3 mL) is calculated assuming a volume expansion coefficient of 100%. The volume of the components making up the mixture is 2 × 29.58 mL or 59.16 mL.
   59.16 mL × 1.095 g/mL = 64.78 grams
3. The caloric content of the total product is also calculated as follows:

Carbohydrates	$[17 \times (10 \times 0.52)] \times 4 = 88.8$
Protein	$(10 \times 0.36) \times 4 = 14.4$
Fat	$16 \times 6 = 144$
Total	247.2

In Table 5.2, the caloric content of several different types of ice cream with varying volume expansion coefficients, calculated using the aforementioned method, is also shown. The caloric values of several other types of ice cream with different nutritional values are also presented in Table 5.3.

Ice cream consumers often request it based on its weight. The figures in the above-mentioned table indicate that various types of ice cream provide 5–10% of the daily energy requirement for an inactive elderly individual (2000 kcal). Different aspects like a balanced and varied diet can also be met through its consumption.

Table 5.2 Caloric content of a serving of different ice cream types (Regarding fat and volume expansion coefficient).

Energy in a 120 g serving (kcal)	Volume expansion coefficient (%)	Weight per serving (g)	Density (g/mL)	Percent		
				Sweeteners[a]	Nonfat solid milk	Fat
160	100	64.8	1.095	17	10	16
240	50	97.2	1.095	17	10	16
119	100	61.6	1.042	17	10	10
179	50	92.4	1.042	17	10	10
105	100	66.2	1.120	17	17	5
158	50	99.3	1.120	17	17	5
91	100	67.9	1.150	22	17	0
136	50	102	1.150	22	17	0

a) Includes maltodextrins, polydextroses, and corn syrup, which cover low-fat or nonfat parts of ice cream.

Table 5.3 Classification of various types of vanilla ice cream based on composition and nutritional value.

Type	Calcium (g)	Sugar (g)	Carbohydrates	Protein	Fat	Calories (kcal)
Fat-Free	10	13	19	3.5	0	90
Low-Fat	9	15	18	3	2.3	100
Half-Fat	9	15	17.2	3	3.3	110
Full-Fat	8	3	13	3	4	100
Regular	8	13	15	2.3	7.2	135
Premium	7	14	17	2.4	9.8	165

5.1.3 Protein Content in Ice Cream

The content of nonfat solid milk in ice cream is substantial, with proteins from milk constituting around 36–34% of it. This milk protein holds a very high "biological value" as it encompasses all "essential amino acids." Milk protein is notably rich in tryptophan and lysine. Protein is a vital element of animal life as it is present in the composition of protoplasm in every living cell. Milk protein is not only a complete protein, but its digestibility after absorption is also approximately 6–5% higher than other proteins, making it nearly complete. The protein content in food is determined by analyzing its nitrogen content. Early protein breakdown studies revealed that proteins contain nearly 16% nitrogen. The general rule for protein determination is to multiply the nitrogen content by a factor of 6/25. For milk protein, this factor is 6.38.

5.1.4 Fat Content in Ice Cream

About 95.8% of the fat in ice cream consists of triglycerides of fatty acids. Triglycerides are compounds where three fatty acids are bonded to a three-carbon alcohol molecule called glycerol through ester linkages. Mono-, di-, and triglycerides, respectively, contain one, two, or three fatty acids in their molecules. Milk fat is uniquely rich in butyric acid (4 carbons) and caproic acid (6 carbons) among fats and oils. In 100 moles of milk fatty acids, 11.8 and 4.6% of butyric acid and caproic acid are present, respectively. All butyric acid and 93% of caproic acid are esterified at the third carbon of glycerol. Milk fat also contains 2.25% diglycerides, 0.08% monoglycerides, 1.11% phospholipids (from nine different types), 0.46% cholesterol, and 0.28% free fatty acids. Although milk fat comprises only 4.5% of "saturated fatty acids," 27% of "monounsaturated fatty acids" are formed by fatty acids with a double bond. The fat content of ice cream is usually determined by extracting and weighing the soluble portion in ether. A significant aspect of milk fat in ice cream pertains to its functional properties. In ice cream, fat serves as an energy source, a supplier of essential fatty acids and fat-soluble vitamins, and carries both saturated and unsaturated fatty acids and sterols such as cholesterol. Fat in ice cream also contributes to its unique flavor. It serves as a solvent for flavor and aroma compounds and also creates a sensation of mouth-coating when consuming ice cream. It plays an effective role in the structure of ice cream and beyond, affecting the texture of ice cream and other frozen desserts.

5.1.5 Carbohydrate Content in Ice Cream

Carbohydrates in ice cream include starch, dextrin, cellulose, sugars, pectins, gums, and their derivatives. Carbohydrates serve as a source of energy and heat production in the body. These compounds are broken down by enzymes secreted in the digestive system into simple sugars, with glucose being the major end product. Several types of sugars can be used in ice cream production. The most commonly used sugar is sucrose, which is a disaccharide. Sucrose is obtained from sugar beets or sugarcane, with no significant difference between the two sources. Corn syrup is also widely used, primarily containing glucose (dextrose) or its modified forms like maltose or fructose (levulose). Fruits typically contain sugars such as sucrose, fructose, and glucose. Invert sugar is a mixture of equal amounts of fructose and glucose monosaccharides, commonly used nowadays. Lactose (milk sugar) is a disaccharide that comprises over a third of milk solids and almost 20% of ice cream carbohydrates. Lactose is unique as it exists only in milk, whereas other sugars are widely found in nature. Many individuals produce a negligible amount of the enzyme lactase in their stomachs, preventing them from hydrolyzing all the lactose present in an ice cream serving. For lactose to be absorbed through the intestinal wall, it needs to be broken down and converted into a monosaccharide. If this does not occur, it can lead to discomfort, including bloating and, in worse cases, diarrhea. These symptoms arise when lactose enters the large intestine and increases osmotic pressure in the environment, causing water to be drawn into the large intestine and resulting in diarrhea. Furthermore, lactose serves as a suitable food substrate for large intestinal bacteria called Coliform. These bacteria ferment lactose, producing gas and acids. The gas generated from lactose fermentation contributes to flatulence. There are four ways to prevent or alleviate the symptoms of incomplete lactose absorption.

The first is for consumers to choose very high-fat ice cream. Higher fat content means less nonfat solid and consequently less lactose. High-fat ice cream is generally more expensive, and its nonfat solid component is usually derived from skim milk powder. Skim milk powder contains 50% less lactose than whey. Nonfat solids from whey can provide over a quarter of the nonfat solid content in ice cream and can be used as a replacement for cheaper ice cream. The second method is to consume ice cream at the end of a meal. In this case, lactose moves relatively slowly through the digestive system, requiring fewer enzymes for hydrolysis and resulting in a lower lactose concentration available to large intestinal bacteria. The third method is consuming yoghurt ice cream. This product contains live yoghurt bacteria that have previously fermented a portion of the lactose during yoghurt preparation. Residual live bacteria present in the ice cream can also release lactase in the human intestine. Freezing, however, destroys about 90% of yoghurt bacteria, and if encapsulated bacteria are used, only about 50% of them will survive freezing. When these bacteria are encapsulated with sodium alginate, they remain viable after freezing. The fourth method to reduce the effects of incomplete lactose absorption is to limit the lactose content in frozen desserts. This can be done by hydrolyzing lactose with beta-galactosidase before freezing. This enzyme is expensive and requires a long time for hydrolysis. Since hydrolyzing each lactose molecule produces two molecules, the freezing point of the mixture might drop considerably.

Moreover, another approach is to separate lactose from skim milk by using membrane separation or ultrafiltration techniques. Separating 50% of the lactose using ultrafiltration and then hydrolyzing the remaining lactose with enzymes will result in a concentrated mixture with the same freezing point as skim milk concentrate containing the same amount of nonfat solids. Digestibility, heat of combustion, and coefficient of digestibility are used to calculate the energy content of milk carbohydrates, with values of 98%, 3.95, and 3.8 kcal/g, respectively.

5.1.6 Mineral Content in Ice Cream

Several inorganic elements are essential for the growth and functioning of the body. The major essential elements include calcium, phosphorus, magnesium, sodium, potassium, and sulfur, referred to as major or abundant minerals. Another category consists of trace minerals, which are required in smaller amounts and include copper, cobalt, iodine, manganese, zinc, fluorine, molybdenum, and selenium, referred to as trace or minor minerals. The major minerals are interdependent and need to be present in specific proportions in the diet. Calcium and phosphorus have essential roles, particularly in building strong bones and teeth and have unique functional roles in dairy products. Over 85% of phosphorus in the body is in combination with calcium, mainly in bones and teeth. Milk and dairy products are rich sources of phosphorus. Almost all the calcium and phosphorus in ice cream are derived from dairy sources, and their amounts are proportional to the nonfat solid content. Since the nonfat solid content in ice cream is about 6–14%, and the calcium content in nonfat solids is about 13.8 mg per gram, a 70-gram serving of ice cream can contain between 135 and 58 mg of calcium. The average value is around 96.5 mg, meeting 8–12% of the recommended daily calcium intake in a person's diet. For children, the recommendation is 800 mg, and for adults, it is 1200 mg per day. Similarly, because every gram of nonfat solid contains about 0.1 mg of phosphorus, a 70-gram serving of ice cream can provide 105–45 mg of phosphorus. The recommended daily intake for phosphorus is 1200 mg for individuals aged 11–24 and 800 mg for others (except infants), making ice cream a significant source of phosphorus. A 70-gram serving of ice cream can provide 10% of the daily phosphorus requirement. Fortunately, milk contains only small amounts of copper and iron. These two minerals catalyze oxidation reactions. Since ice cream can be stored for weeks or even months after production before consumption, it is essential to prevent the contamination of its components with these minerals. This is also the primary reason why equipment used in dairy production is designed to minimize copper contact.

5.1.7 Vitamins in Ice Cream

Ice cream, like milk, is also an important source of several vitamins, and its content depends on the amount of nonfat solids in milk and the weight of the ice cream. Fat-soluble vitamins such as A, D, E, and K are primarily soluble in fat, and products enriched with nonfat components are devoid of these vitamins. Milk fat is a good source of vitamin A. Therefore, ice cream producers need to add vitamin A to their low-fat or nonfat products. The amount of water-soluble vitamins in regular ice cream is proportional to the amount of nonfat solid in milk. In nonfat ice creams, the content of these vitamins is higher, and in high-fat ice creams, it is at its lowest. Some of these water-soluble vitamins in ice cream come from fruits and nuts. Ice cream is a good source of riboflavin. Similar to what was mentioned about calcium, a 70-gram serving of ice cream provides 10% of the individual's riboflavin requirement. The amount of riboflavin is 18 mg per gram of nonfat solid milk and 175–75 micrograms in a 70-gram serving of ice cream. Ice cream also contains significant amounts of thiamine, pyridoxine (vitamin B6), and pantothenic acid. These vitamins play important roles in various physiological processes in the body, contributing to overall health and well-being. It is essential to note that the vitamin content in ice cream can vary depending on the specific recipe and ingredients used by manufacturers.

5.1.8 Digestibility of Ice Cream

The digestibility of ice cream is one of the important factors in choosing it as a desirable food. Many flavoring and aromatic ingredients can be incorporated into ice cream. Ice cream does not require chewing and its soft and smooth texture satisfies the sense of taste. The coldness of ice cream makes it a desirable food, especially in hot weather. Ice cream is generally highly digestible. The incomplete lactose absorption in some individuals is an exception in terms of the nutritional value of ice cream. However, the symptoms resulting from incomplete lactose absorption for a serving of ice cream are not significant compared to consuming a cup of milk a day. Therefore, even when there is no demand for other food items, ice cream remains an ideal food. No other food with this level of nutritional value is as appealing and beloved by the general public. In summary, ice cream is a food that is not only delicious but also provides essential nutrients and offers a pleasurable eating experience. Its smooth texture and cooling nature make it a popular choice, especially during warm weather. The combination of fats, sugars, proteins, minerals, and vitamins in ice cream creates a unique and enjoyable treat that has captured the hearts of people worldwide (Marshall et al. 2003).

References

Homayouni, A. (2008). Effect of microencapsulation and resistant starch on the probiotic survival and sensory properties of synbiotic ice cream. PhD Thesis. University of Tehran, Iran.

Marshall, R.T., Goff, H.D., and Hartel, R.W. (2003). *Ice cream*, 6e. New York: Kluwer Academic/Plenum Publishers. 371pp.

Part II

The Technology of Probiotic Ice Cream

6

Probiotic Ice Cream (Definition, Formulation, and Characterization)

6.1 Definition of Probiotic Ice Cream

Probiotic ice cream refers to ice cream containing live microbial cells (probiotics) that can be produced through either fermentation or nonfermentation methods, based on dairy, soy milk, and other plant-based proteins. Probiotics can be used in free form or microencapsulated in ice cream formulations. Probiotics are live microorganisms that, when consumed in sufficient amounts and in their live form, can exert health-promoting effects on the host. Ice cream has a good distribution capability for probiotics among consumers. Studies have explored the possibility of adding probiotics to both fermented and nonfermented ice creams. Among lactic acid bacteria, *Lactobacillus* and *Bifidobacterium* species are commonly used as suitable probiotics in the production of fermented dairy products. In frozen dairy products, ice cream has received attention due to its near-neutral pH (around 7), which provides favorable conditions for enhancing the viability of probiotic bacteria. The high dry matter content of ice cream contributes to the protection and viability of probiotic bacteria. However, the viability of probiotics is influenced by factors such as the type of dairy product, the presence of air, and the storage temperature. Probiotic bacteria must be resistant to the production and storage conditions as well as the harsh conditions of the digestive system. Live probiotic bacteria have greater therapeutic effects compared to nonliving cells or cell components. Therefore, the International Dairy Federation recommends a minimum of 10^7 (ten million) live bacteria per gram of dairy product for therapeutic effects at time of consumption. However, studies have shown that the viability of probiotics in frozen dairy products faces challenges unless suitable methods are employed to prevent potential damage during freezing and the presence of oxygen. Improving the viability of probiotics depends on the type of food product. Selecting probiotic strains resistant to production and

Probiotic Ice Cream: Science and Technology, First Edition. Aziz Homayouni-Rad.

storage conditions, as well as gastrointestinal conditions, and altering processing and storage conditions, are among the strategies considered. Direct protection of probiotics through microencapsulation is another method to enhance their viability. Microencapsulation separates probiotic cells from unfavorable food and digestive system conditions, thereby increasing their shelf life in frozen dairy products. In conclusion, microencapsulation is a novel method for directly protecting probiotics, preventing the adverse effects on food and the gastrointestinal system, and increasing their shelf life in frozen dairy products (Homayouni 2008).

6.2 Design of Probiotic Ice Cream

The development of probiotic ice cream is a complex endeavor that demands a deep understanding of both the product itself and the preferences and needs of the consumers. It also necessitates effective management of customer knowledge. From a research and development perspective, creating functional probiotic ice cream requires collaboration across various fields, including food technology, nutrition, medicine, and food chemistry. The goal is to produce innovative products that can positively impact physiological parameters related to health and disease prevention. The design and development of functional probiotic ice cream is a multifaceted and costly process. It involves the consideration of numerous factors, such as sensory appeal, physicochemical and microbial stability, pricing, and other inherent functional properties, all of which are essential for success in the market. Furthermore, it is crucial to align these products with consumer expectations regarding functional probiotic products. So, the creation of probiotic ice cream is a holistic endeavor that merges scientific expertise, consumer insights, and innovative product development to deliver not only a tasty treat but also potential health benefits. This interdisciplinary approach is essential for meeting both market demands and consumer expectations. Nowadays two types of probiotic ice cream have been designed and formulated in frozen and shake forms (Homayouni 2008).

6.3 Probiotic Ice Cream Characterization

Numerous investigations have been conducted to assess the suitability of ice cream as a vehicle for delivery of probiotics. These studies primarily focused on evaluating the taste and sensory acceptability of these products and their ability to preserve the viability of bacteria. Several studies explored the use of probiotics alone in ice cream to determine their effectiveness as a probiotic carrier. The initial study utilized strains including *Lactobacillus acidophilus* and *Bifidobacterium bifidum*. Sensory results were positive, although bacterial counts decreased over the 90-day storage period, they still retained their probiotic qualities. In contrast, a second study indicated that ice cream alone was less effective in preserving bacteria viability. However, when ice cream incorporated prebiotics like fructooligosaccharide (FOS) or inulin, these ingredients aided in maintaining bacterial viability. Both studies involved inoculating a portion of the milk and later adding it to the rest of the ingredients after cooling. Studies demonstrated that probiotic bacteria survived the freezing process when incorporated into ice cream making it a probiotic food carrier. The sensory characteristics of a synbiotic ice cream in which sucrose was substituted with either inulin or FOS at levels of 10, 20, or 30% were investigated. The ice cream formulations included the probiotic species *L. casei KE99* (0.3 g) and *Bifidobacterium bifidum* (0.3g). These probiotics were purchased as freeze-dried cultures and were labeled as 100% pure and food-grade. Results indicated that the 30% FOS negatively impacted flavor and texture, while the addition of inulin did not affect sweetness, smoothness, flavor, texture, or overall acceptability of the ice cream. Furthermore, the inclusion of probiotics had no significant impact on the sensory attributes of the ice cream samples. Another study examined the viability of probiotics during ice cream storage revealing that *L. casei KE99* and *Bifidobacterium bifidum* remained viable over a four-month period (120 days), making these bacteria suitable choices for probiotic and synbiotic ice cream. Recent investigations explored the use of microencapsulation to evaluate its impact on bacterial survival within synbiotic ice cream. All studies reported a slower reduction in probiotic bacteria over the storage period. The most favorable results were achieved when microencapsulated bacteria were incorporated into chocolate particles. Overall, microencapsulation was found to be an effective method for maintaining probiotic viability within ice cream (Homayouni 2008).

6.4 Technology of Probiotic Ice Cream Production

Probiotic ice cream and frozen yoghurt are products that can be produced today. Studies have shown that the probiotics present in ice cream do not undergo significant changes during one year of frozen storage. Frozen yoghurt provides a stable environment for the survival and delivery of probiotics. Regular and fermented ice creams have good distribution capabilities among consumers. The low storage temperature of frozen dairy products provides ideal conditions for the long-term viability of probiotic bacteria. Fermented dairy desserts made from yoghurt have a low pH (around 4.5 or lower), which reduces the viability of live bacteria like *Lactobacillus acidophilus* and *Bifidobacterium* species due to the low pH. However, adding probiotic bacteria to ice cream does not pose a problem because the pH in ice cream (around 5.6–6.6) is ideal for their viability. The only challenge is air incorporation during freezing, which affects the viability of probiotics due to the presence of oxygen. The microencapsulation of probiotic bacteria in ice cream can prevent the toxic effects of oxygen on these bacteria. This approach can maintain their viability and effectiveness (Homayouni 2008). Another way is to substitute the air with nitrogen gas in aeration of ice cream. Crystallization of lactose in ice cream may occur due to the higher solubility of sucrose and the consequent concentration of lactose in the nonfrozen portion, especially under low-temperature conditions. This situation can potentially lead to damage to the cell walls of probiotics and changes in the permeability of cell membranes. In formulation of premium ice cream, conditions are set in such a way that the possibility of lactose crystallization and the occurrence of a gritty texture are eliminated. To better comprehend the subject, let us first distinguish between "grittiness" and "roughness" of the texture of ice cream. Roughness is the predominant defect observed in ice cream texture, resulting from the growth of ice crystals during storage. The size of ice crystals approximately doubles after 200 days of storage. However, the grittiness of the texture arises from the crystallization of alpha-lactose monohydrate in ice cream, especially after freezing, when lactose in the nonfrozen portion becomes concentrated. Lactose crystals can be distinguished from ice crystals by their slower solubility rate. To prevent lactose crystallization, its concentration is reduced in the formulation, and temperature fluctuations are avoided. Typically, when the lactose concentration in the formulation is less than 2%, lactose crystallization reaches its minimum level, and gritty texture is not noticeable. In the formulation of premium ice cream, the lactose concentration is less than 2%, thus avoiding the occurrence of a gritty texture. To prevent texture roughening due to water crystallization, increasing solid ingredients, adding suitable stabilizers, rapid freezing, and sharpening freezer blades can be taken. In fact, prebiotic-resistant starch in premium ice cream formulation significantly prevents texture roughening and ensures a smooth texture. Grittiness of the texture often occurs in retailers' freezers due to temperature fluctuations, which accelerate lactose crystallization. In cases where the use of nonfat dry milk with high lactose content (containing around 50% lactose) is required in the formulation (for ice cream containing 18–16% serum solids), adding a portion of it after the mixture has slightly thickened during freezing can prevent grittiness.

In this scenario, the mechanism works as follows: In semifrozen ice cream, the nonfrozen portion becomes saturated with lactose. As a result, the anhydrous lactose present in nonfat dry milk, which cannot dissolve in the nonfrozen part of the ice cream inside the freezer, cannot contribute to grittiness. Additionally, due to the high number of small-sized lactose crystals in nonfat dry milk, even after water absorption and crystallization, they cannot create a gritty texture. By substituting a portion of sucrose with corn syrup and using an appropriate stabilizer like locust bean gum, conditions are made unfavorable for lactose crystallization, and the increased viscosity prevents lactose crystallization. Therefore, the type and amount of stabilizer play a crucial role in preventing grittiness (Homayouni 2008). For the formulation of probiotic ice cream, the following ingredients can be used: skim milk, heavy cream (40% fat), dry milk, sucrose, stabilizer, emulsifier, flavoring (vanillin), and resistant starch. To produce probiotic ice cream, the equipment to be used (a double-walled agitated tank as a formulation and pasteurization tank, and a homogenizer) is thoroughly cleaned and sanitized. Then, the ice cream ingredients, which have been preweighed, are mixed together in the following sequence:

1. Skim milk and heavy cream are added to the formulation tank and gently heated. When the temperature reaches 50°C, nonfat dry milk and resistant starch, mixed with half of the sucrose, are added slowly. The other half of the sucrose is mixed with stabilizer and emulsifier. Once the temperature reaches 60°C, this mixture is added to the formulation tank.
2. Heating continues until reaching 70°C, and the resulting mixture is kept at 70°C for 30 minutes to be pasteurized. During this time, while the agitator is active, flavoring agents are added.
3. The ice cream mixture is then subjected to a two-stage homogenization process in a homogenizer, first at 170 bar and then at 40 bar. The mixture is cooled to 4°C and held at this temperature for 12 hours to allow the mixture to mature.
4. Afterward, either free or microencapsulated probiotic cells are added to the nonfermented probiotic ice cream. Immediately after adding the probiotics, the mixture is frozen in a freezer with an overrun of 100%, and then it is packaged in 100-gram cups and transferred to −20°C as shown in Figure 6.1.

6.5 Adding Free and Microencapsulated Probiotic Bacteria into the Ice Cream

Probiotic bacteria, including *L. casei* and *B. lactis*, in both free and microencapsulated forms, are immediately added to the ice cream mixture before

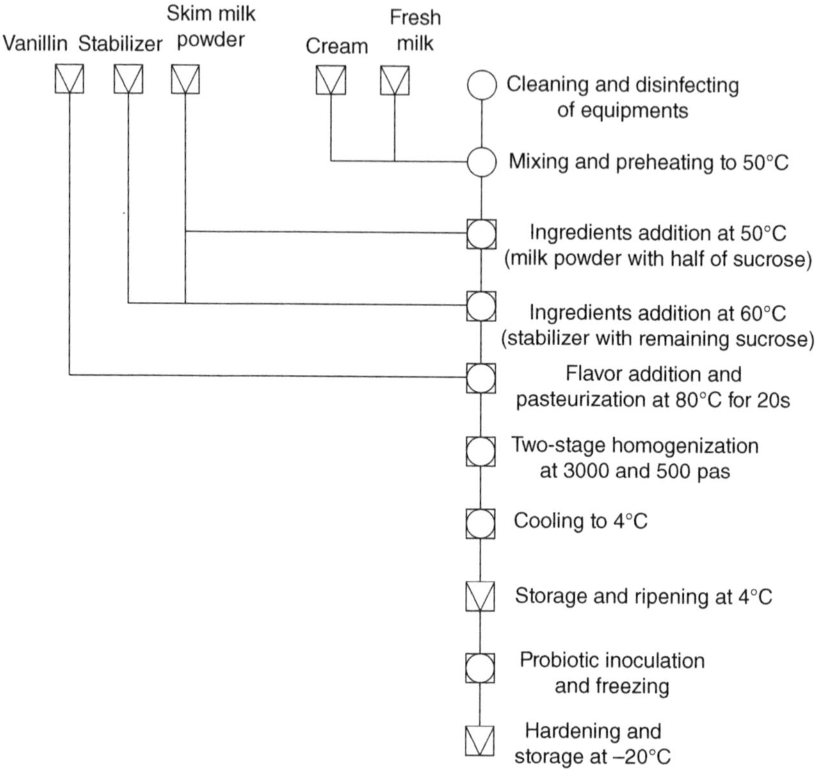

Figure 6.1 Probiotic ice cream production process (Homayouni et al. 2008) / with permission of Elsevier.

freezing. In a study, five types of ice cream were prepared: the first type contained free *L. casei* cells, the second type contained microencapsulated *L. casei* cells, the third type contained free *B. lactis* cells, the fourth type contained microencapsulated *B. lactis* cells, and the fifth type of ice cream was devoid of both free and microencapsulated cells, serving as the control. In the formulation of all ice cream types, 1% starch was used. The number of live bacteria in the ice cream mixture before freezing of ice cream was 10^9 colony forming unit (CFU) per gram. The results showed that microencapsulated bacteria tend to remain more viable compared to free cells. Furthermore, after six months of storage at −20°C, microencapsulated *B. lactis* showed higher viability compared to microencapsulated *L. casei*. Figures 6.2 and 6.3 illustrate the number of live bacteria in the initial ice cream mixture and in the final product during six months of storage at −20°C, both before and after freezing. The reduction in the number of live

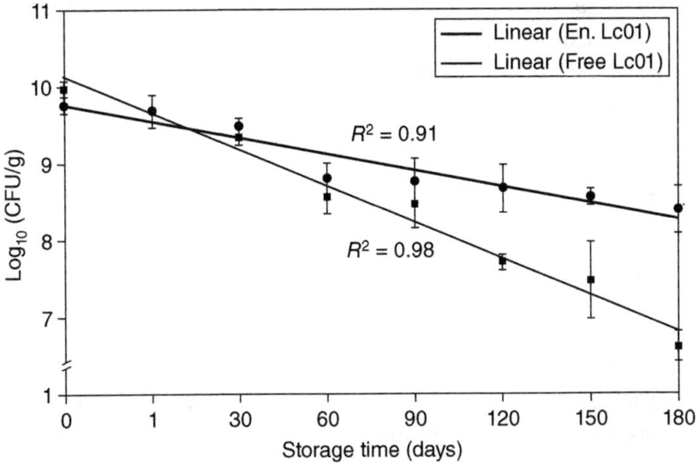

Figure 6.2 Survival of free and encapsulated *L. casei (Lc-01)* cells in probiotic ice cream during 180 days of storage at −20°C. Error bars indicate standard error (Homayouni et al. 2008) / with permission of Elsevier.

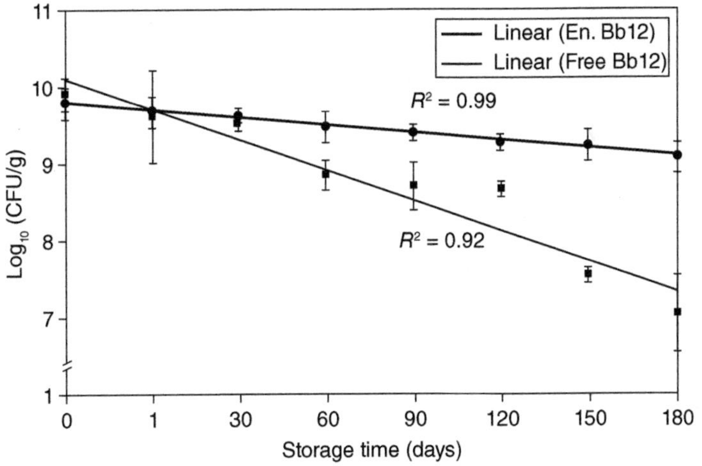

Figure 6.3 Survival of free and encapsulated *B. lactis (Bb-12)* cells in probiotic ice cream during 180 days of storage at −20°C. Error bars indicate standard error (Homayouni et al. 2008) / with permission of Elsevier.

L. casei and *B. lactis*, whether in free or microencapsulated form, shows a statistically significant difference. Therefore, it can be concluded that the viability of probiotic bacteria depends on the type of bacteria and its form (free or encapsulated).

References

Homayouni, A. (2008). Effect of microencapsulation and resistant starch on the probiotic survival and sensory properties of synbiotic ice cream. PhD thesis, University of Tehran, Iran.

Homayouni, A., Azizi, A., Ehsani, M.R., and Yarmand, M.S. (2008). Effect of microencapsulation and resistant starch on the probiotic survival and sensory properties of synbiotic ice cream. *Food Chemistry* 111 (1): 50–55.

7

Prebiotic Ice Cream (Definition, Formulation, and Characterization)

7.1 Definition of Prebiotic Ice Cream

Prebiotic ice cream is a type of ice cream that contains prebiotic compounds. Prebiotics are substances that promote the growth and activity of beneficial microorganisms in the gut. When included in ice cream, prebiotics can have a positive impact on gut health. Prebiotics are nondigestible or poorly digestible carbohydrates that, upon reaching the gut environment, selectively stimulate the growth and activity of probiotics. When such food enters the large intestine, prebiotics are consumed by probiotics and enhance their population, leading to a decrease in the population of pathogenic bacteria (Homayouni 2009).

7.2 Prebiotics

Prebiotics are nondigestible or partially digestible oligosaccharides that, upon reaching the intestinal environment, selectively promote the growth or activity of probiotics. Prebiotic compounds exist in two natural and artificial categories. For many years, prebiotics have been a part of the human diet. However, in the 1990s, the importance of prebiotics in regulating the gut bacteria ratio was discovered. The term "prebiotic" was first introduced by Gibson and Roberfroid in 1995. Nowadays, prebiotics refer to food components that selectively alter the gut bacteria's composition and activity, promoting the host's health. Recently, scientists have been paying more attention to prebiotics than probiotics, and extensive research is underway in this field. It seems that prebiotics may be more important than probiotics because each individual has their own specific probiotics, and these bacteria vary from one region to another worldwide. Therefore, it is better to develop

Probiotic Ice Cream: Science and Technology, First Edition. Aziz Homayouni-Rad.

the digestive system's specific probiotics rather than introducing new probiotic species into the human body, either pure or within food products. This can easily be achieved through prebiotics (Homayouni 2009).

7.2.1 Classifications of Prebiotics

Prebiotics are typically carbohydrates (sugars) that remain undigested and unabsorbed in the human small intestine. As a result, they enter the large intestine in their original form and become available for consumption by probiotics. On the other hand, probiotics are saccharolytic (sugar-fermenting) in nature. This is why complex carbohydrates that enter the large intestine only reach probiotics' consumption, leading to an increased population of these bacteria compared to other bacteria. Prebiotic carbohydrates can be categorized into two groups: oligosaccharides (2–20 monomer units) and polysaccharides (more than 20 monomer units). Oligosaccharides include lactulose, lactosaccharides, isomalto-oligosaccharides, gluco-oligosaccharides, fructo-oligosaccharides (FOS), galacto-oligosaccharides, soy oligosaccharides, and human milk oligosaccharides. Resistant starch and dietary fiber are polysaccharide prebiotics. The physicochemical properties of nondigestible carbohydrates make them suitable replacements for simple sugars in foods. Today, these carbohydrates are used in food production for various purposes, such as reducing sweetness in foods, increasing viscosity, lowering freezing point, and slowing down Maillard reactions in products. Additionally, the physiological characteristics of nondigestible carbohydrates, such as being low in calories and having a low glycemic index, are of significant importance. These attributes have led to the widespread use of these carbohydrates in the production of various food products, including ice cream, yoghurt, fruit juices, bread, and confectionery products. In the next sections, the mentioned prebiotics will be discussed (Homayouni 2009).

7.2.1.1 Lactulose

Lactose is used as the primary material for the production of lactulose and lactosaccharides (see Figure 7.1). Alkaline isomerization leads to the conversion of the glucose portion of lactulose into fructose, resulting in lactulose (4-oxo-beta-galactopyranosyl-d-fructose), which is indigestible in the human gut. In the field of medicine, lactulose has long been produced for the treatment of constipation and hepatitis. The lack of digestion of lactulose by digestive system enzymes causes it to enter the large intestine in its original form, where it is consumed by the microbiota of the large intestine, especially bifidobacteria. Compounds like this, which enhance

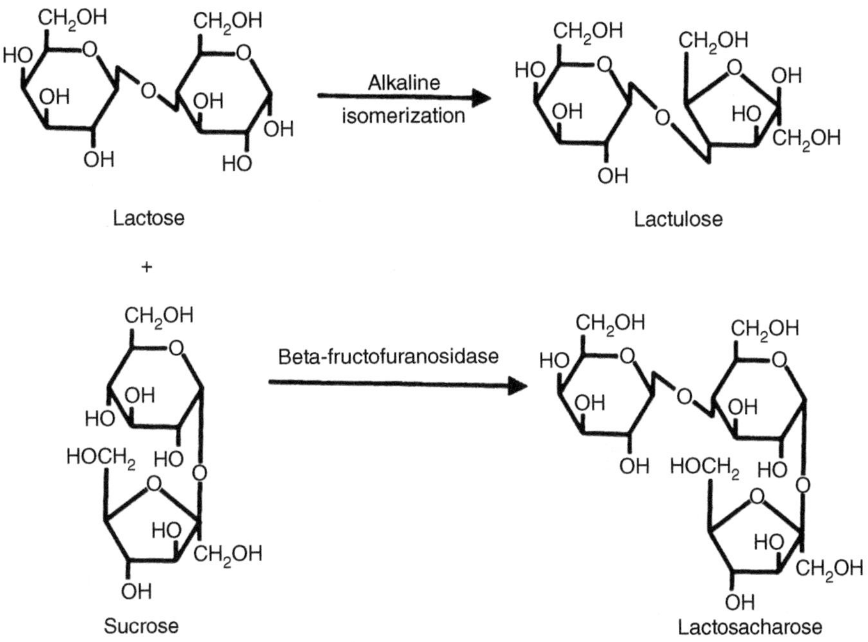

Figure 7.1 Lactulose and lactosaccharose made from lactose.

the growth or activity of bifidobacteria, are referred to as bifidogenic compounds or bifidus factors. Lactulose was the first bifidogenic compound recognized for its positive effect on the growth of bifidobacteria in 1957. Similar to fructans and galactans, it promotes the growth of probiotics in the human intestine and reduces the number of Bacteroides, streptococci, *Clostridium perfringens*, and enterobacteria without causing flatulence or bloating. Due to its prebiotic effects, lactulose is consumed as a dietary component in Japan and is widely used in the production of various foods and beverages. The mechanism of action of lactulose in preventing the growth of pathogenic bacteria in the intestine is attributed to acidifying the intestinal environment due to its rapid fermentation (Homayouni 2009).

7.2.1.2 Lactosaccharose

Lactosaccharose is a nondigestible trisaccharide in the human body that is produced from lactose and sucrose (see Figure 7.1). Its chemical structure is beta-d-galactopyranosyl-(1→4)-alpha-d-glucopyranosyl-beta-d-fructofuranoside. The conversion of lactose and sucrose into lactosaccharide is carried out by the enzyme beta-fructofuranosidase. Lactosaccharide is commonly used in beverages, confectionery products, and sugar cubes.

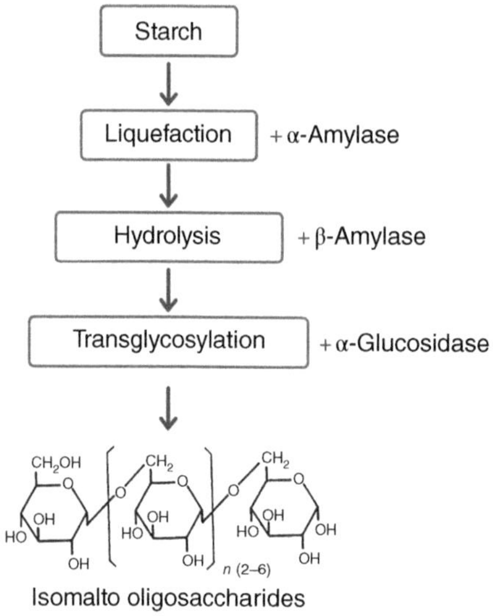

Figure 7.2 Production of isomalto-oligosaccharides from starch.

Lactosaccharide is also capable of increasing the population of bifidobacteria in the human large intestine (Homayouni 2009).

7.2.1.3 Isomalto-oligosaccharides

Isomalto-oligosaccharides are formed from starch in a two-step reaction. In the first step, starch is liquefied by the enzyme alpha-amylase. Then, it is converted into isomalto-oligosaccharides by the action of beta-amylase and alpha-glucosidase, which contain molecules with alpha (1→6) and alpha (1→4) glucose residues with a polymerization degree of 6–2 (see Figure 7.2). Although some isomalto-oligosaccharides are digested and absorbed unlike other prebiotics when passing through the digestive system, some of them still enter the large intestine undigested and exert bifidogenic effects. Consumption of 10–20 grams of isomalto-oligosaccharides per day specifically increases the population of bifidobacteria and plays a positive role in the treatment of constipation and lowering of harmful serum cholesterol (Homayouni 2009).

7.2.1.4 Xylo-oligo-saccharides

Xylo-oligo-saccharides (XOS) are produced from xylans derived from corn residues. In this process, xylans are hydrolyzed by the enzyme endo-1, 4-beta-xylanase, and xylose monosaccharides, along with high molecular weight carbohydrates, are separated by fractionation and reverse osmosis. The remaining carbohydrates are primarily XOS connected to each other by beta-(1→4) linkages, including xylobiose, xylotriose, and xylotetraose.

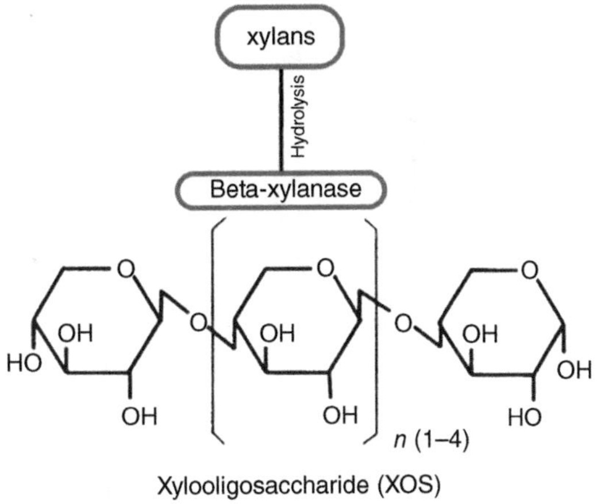

Figure 7.3 Production of xylo-oligo-saccharides from xylan.

In this process, some branched oligosaccharides with arabinose side branches are also produced (see Figure 7.3). XOS selectively enhance the growth of bifidobacteria. Their efficiency in increasing the population of bifidobacteria is even greater when compared to FOS (Homayouni 2009).

7.2.1.5 Fructo-oligosaccharides

Fructo-oligosaccharides (FOS) and inulin (see Figure 7.4) are also undigested in the human stomach and small intestine, entering the large intestine undigested, where they promote the growth of species like *Bifidobacterium*, *Lactobacillus*, and *Eubacterium*. The increase in the number of *Clostridium cocoides* and *Eubacterium rectale* bacteria leads to an increase in butyrate production and a decrease in pH in the large intestine. Inulin is found in many fruits and vegetables and has been used by humans for thousands of years. Today, inulin and FOS are produced as white, odorless powders. FOS are also available as thick syrups with a concentration of 75% (by weight). Inulin is used as a fat replacer and emulsion stabilizer in ice cream, improving mouth feel and the freezing point of the ice cream. FOS and inulin are used in frozen desserts, yoghurt, cheese, various types of bread, biscuits, chocolates, and meat products in addition to ice cream and dietetic products (Homayouni 2009).

7.2.1.6 Galacto-oligosaccharides

Galacto-oligosaccharides are nondigestible carbohydrates in the human body that are produced from lactose by the enzyme beta-galactosidase (Figure 7.5) and are found in human milk at a concentration of one gram per liter. They are also present in small amounts in cow's milk. These compounds are not digested by digestive enzymes and, after reaching

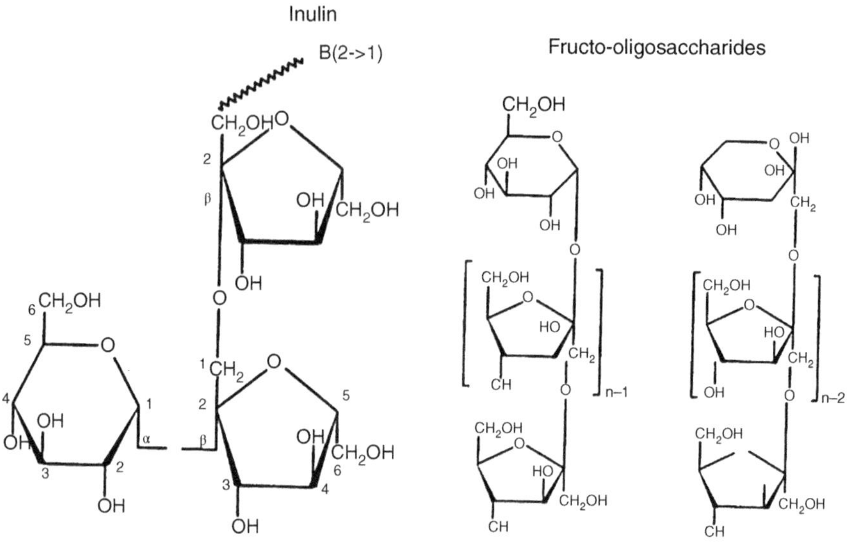

Figure 7.4 Chemical structure of fructo-oligosaccharides and inulin.

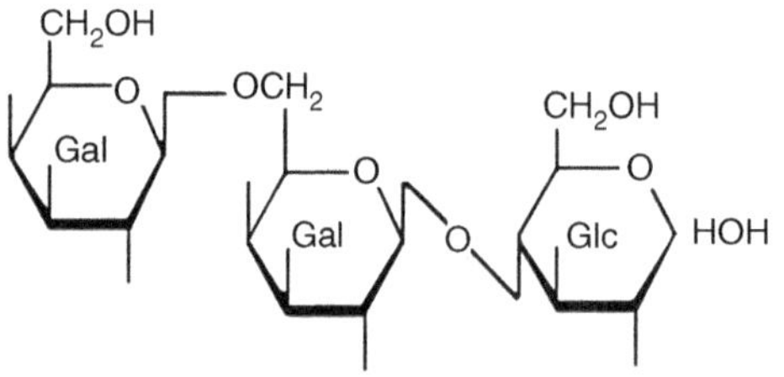

Figure 7.5 Chemical structure of galacto-oligosaccharides.

the large intestine, are consumed by intestinal microbiota, enhancing the growth and activity of probiotics. Human milk galacto-oligosaccharides have a protective role against pathogenic bacteria in infants up to one year of age. Scientists believe that the chemical structure of these compounds bears a strong resemblance to sugar compounds attached to the surface of human intestinal cells, to which pathogenic bacteria adhere through these sugars. In fact, these compounds act as receptors for bacterial cells and bind to pathogenic bacteria, then eliminate them. Galacto-oligosaccharides are soluble in water and exhibit high resistance to heat and acidic conditions. Their sweetness level is approximately 35% compared to sucrose. The use of these sugars in ice cream reduces the freezing point and helps preserve the free water of the product without converting it to ice crystals. They also improve the texture and mouth feel of ice cream. Galacto-oligosaccharides in the human intestine have a prebiotic effect, aiding in the treatment

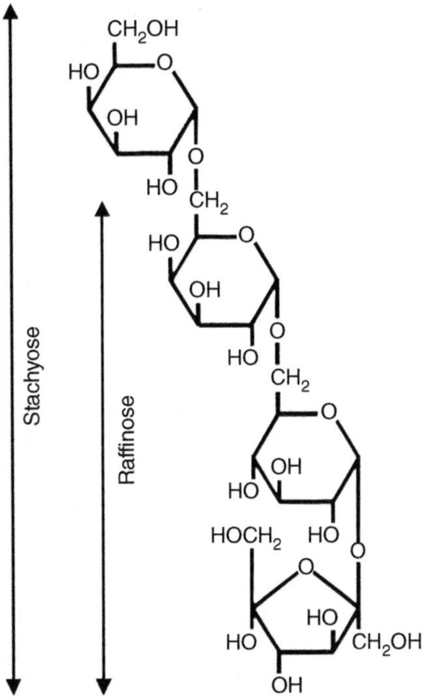

Figure 7.6 Chemical structure of soy oligosaccharides.

of constipation and reducing the activity of enzymes that convert procarcinogenic compounds into carcinogenic ones (Homayouni 2009).

7.2.1.7 Soy Oligosaccharides

Soy oligosaccharides are primarily composed of the trisaccharides raffinose and stachyose (Figure 7.6), which are extracted from the by-products of soy milk production plants. Raffinose and stachyose are resistant to digestion and, as a result, enter the large intestine undigested, where they promote the growth of beneficial bacteria. Additionally, they help strengthen the body's immune system, preventing allergies in consumers (Homayouni 2009).

7.2.1.8 Resistant Starch

Resistant starch is considered a type of polysaccharide prebiotic that may be added to ice cream formulation and undergoes slow fermentation in the colon. It offers several advantages over smaller-molecule prebiotics such as lactulose and nondigestible oligosaccharides. One of these advantages is that consumers can tolerate higher doses of resistant starch in their diet without experiencing flatulence or stomach discomfort due to excessive gas production, damage to the intestinal mucosal layer caused by rapid acid production, or diarrhea resulting from the consumption of high concentrations of small-molecule carbohydrates. The most important characteristic of polysaccharide prebiotics, like resistant starch, is that they provide a constant source of fermentable carbohydrates in the large intestine, preventing colorectal cancer in the rectum and distal colon. These two regions of the large intestine are known to be associated with many human diseases. All of the starch that enters the body with food remains undigested in the small intestine and, as a result, a portion of it enters the large intestine. Resistant starch, which is resistant to enzymatic hydrolysis in the human intestine, can be divided into four types:

1. Physically inaccessible starch found in intact grain kernels or minimally milled grains.
2. Natural granule starch found in foods like potatoes, bananas, and corn.
3. Retrograded starch that forms during processing.
4. Chemically modified starch produced through methods like esterification and etherification or by creating side-chain modifications.

The degree of resistance to digestion in the small intestine and the availability of bacterial fermentation in the large intestine depends on the structure and source of the resistant starch. Resistant starch acts as a butyrogenic prebiotic in the large intestine, making it increase the production of butyric acid in the colon while reducing colon Ph. Animal model studies have shown that resistant starch stimulates the growth of bifidobacteria and lactobacilli. Since a wide spectrum of bacteria in the large intestine possesses amylolytic (starch-digesting) activity, it cannot be claimed that the effect of resistant starch on promoting the growth of probiotics is exclusive. In other words, resistant starch may also be consumed by other amylolytic bacteria. Nevertheless, the production of butyric acid resulting from the fermentation of resistant starch is considered a significant factor in many beneficial effects, such as preventing colorectal cancer. In summary, resistant starch is a polysaccharide prebiotic that provides a constant source of fermentable carbohydrates in the large intestine and has various health benefits, including colorectal cancer prevention (Homayouni 2009).

7.2.1.9 Dietary Fiber

Dietary fiber is another type of polysaccharide prebiotic that, due to its resistance to digestion and absorption in the small intestine, enters the large intestine and undergoes fermentation by probiotics. Cereals are rich sources of dietary fiber, such as beta-glucans and arabinoxylans, which are fermentable by microbiota in the large intestine. Beta-glucan is a branched glucose polymer with beta(1→3) and beta(1→4) bounds. Arabinoxylan is also a polymer of beta-d-xylose with beta(1→4) linkages, and it has alpha-arabinose residues as side branches. *Bifidobacterium bifidum* and *Bifidobacterium adolescentis* are capable of fermenting arabinoxylans under certain conditions. In contrast, pathogenic bacteria like *Escherichia coli*, *C. perfringens*, and *Clostridium difficile* are unable to ferment dietary fiber. The bifidogenic effects of arabinoxylans have been demonstrated in animal studies. Additionally, the consumption of arabinoxylans found in oats has been shown to prevent bloating and abdominal distension in humans. In summary, dietary fiber is a polysaccharide prebiotic that can be added to ice cream formulation and resists digestion in the small intestine, entering the large intestine, where it is fermented by probiotic bacteria, providing various health benefits (Homayouni 2009).

7.3 Design of Prebiotic Ice Cream

Ice cream has a good distribution capability for prebiotics among consumers. Studies have explored the possibility of adding prebiotics to both ice cream matrix and as wall materials in encapsulation of probiotics. Among prebiotics, Inulin and resistant starch are commonly used as suitable prebiotics in ice cream formulation (Homayouni et al. 2008).

7.4 Prebiotic Ice Cream Characterization

In order to assess the consumer acceptance of ice cream enriched with prebiotic ingredients, a commercial ice cream mix was prepared, replacing varying percentages (0, 10, 20, or 30%) of sugar with either FOS or inulin. Participants provided ratings for sensory attributes such as sweetness, smoothness, and vanilla flavor in the prebiotic ice cream. Results indicated that when comparing 10 and 20% inulin ice cream to the control (0% substitution), no significant differences were observed in terms of sweetness, smoothness, vanilla flavor, or overall acceptability ($P < 0.05$). However, the 30% inulin ice cream was notably less sweet than the control and 10 and 20% inulin ice creams. Additionally, the 30% inulin variant exhibited reduced smoothness, diminished vanilla flavor, and lowered overall acceptability compared to both the control and the 10% inulin ice cream ($P < 0.05$). In the case of 10 and 20% FOS ice cream, no significant differences were noted in sweetness, smoothness, vanilla flavor, or overall acceptability when compared to the control ($P < 0.05$). These findings suggest that FOS and inulin may be substituted for up to 20% of the sucrose in prebiotic ice cream (Homayouni 2008).

7.5 Technology of Prebiotic Ice Cream Production

Prebiotic ice cream is a product that can be produced today. Resistant starch and inulin are often used as prebiotic ingredients as well as for substituting the sucrose and fat content in low-calorie (low-sugar and low-fat) ice creams. Studies have shown that the prebiotics present in ice cream do not undergo significant changes during one year of frozen storage. For the formulation of prebiotic ice cream, the following ingredients can be used: skim milk, heavy cream (40% fat), dry milk, sugar, stabilizer, emulsifier, flavoring (vanillin), and resistant starch. To produce prebiotic ice cream, the equipment to be used (a double-walled agitated tank as a formulation and pasteurization tank, and a homogenizer) is thoroughly cleaned and sanitized. Then, the ice cream ingredients, which have been preweighed, are mixed together in the following sequence (Figure 7.7):

1. Skim milk and heavy cream are added to the formulation tank and gently heated. When the temperature reaches 50°C, nonfat dry milk and

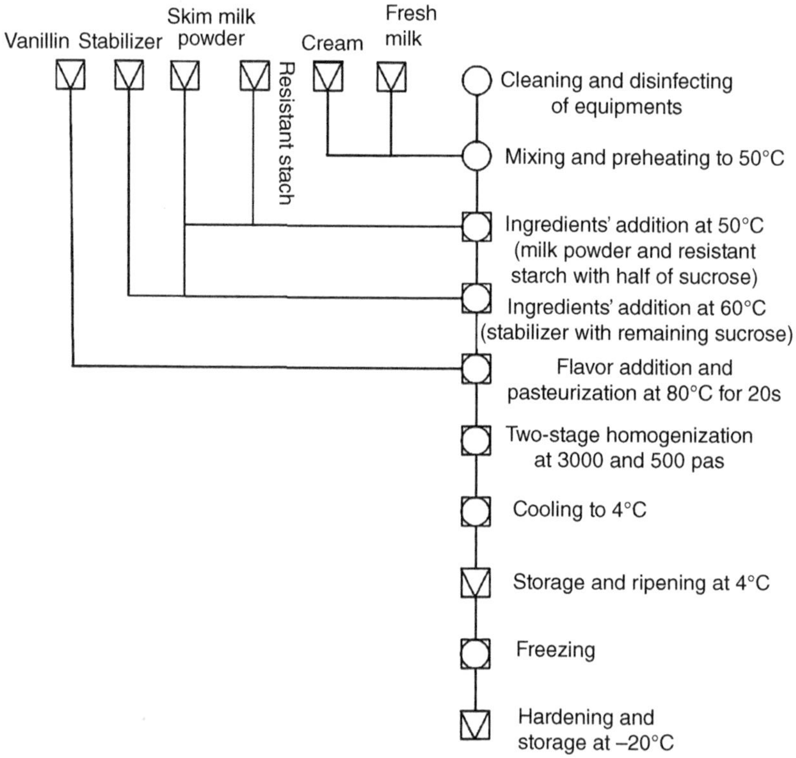

Figure 7.7 Prebiotic ice cream production process (Homayouni et al. 2008) / with permission of Elsevier.

resistant starch, mixed with half of the sucrose, are added slowly. The other half of the sucrose is mixed with stabilizer and emulsifier. Once the temperature reaches 60°C, this mixture is added to the formulation tank.

2. Heating continues until reaching 70°C, and the resulting mixture is kept at 70°C for 30 minutes to be pasteurized. During this time, while the agitator is active, flavoring agents are added.
3. The ice cream mixture is then subjected to a two-stage homogenization process in a homogenizer, first at 170 bar and then at 40 bar. The mixture is cooled to 4°C and held at this temperature for 12 hours to allow the mixture to mature.
4. Afterward, the mixture is frozen in a freezer with an overrun of 100%, and then it is packaged in 100-gram cups and transferred to −20°C.

References

Homayouni, A. (2008). Effect of microencapsulation and resistant starch on the probiotic survival and sensory properties of synbiotic ice cream. PhD thesis, University of Tehran, Iran.

Homayouni, A. (2009). *Therapeutical Effects of Functional Probiotic, Prebiotic and Synbiotic Foods*. Tabriz, Iran: Tabriz University of Medical Sciences.

Homayouni, A., Azizi, A., Ehsani, M.R., and Yarmand, M.S. (2008). Effect of microencapsulation and resistant starch on the probiotic survival and sensory properties of synbiotic ice cream. *Food Chemistry* 111 (1): 50–55.

8

Synbiotic Ice Cream (Definition, Formulation, and Characterization)

8.1 Definition of Synbiotic Ice Cream

Synbiotic ice cream is a formulation where both probiotics and prebiotic components are used simultaneously. This combination aims to provide a synergistic effect by promoting the growth of beneficial microorganisms (probiotics) using prebiotic compounds (Homayouni 2009). The goal of synbiotics is to enhance the overall health benefits of the ice cream. Probiotics are live microorganisms that, when consumed in sufficient amounts and in their live form, exert health-promoting effects on the host. Prebiotics are nondigestible or poorly digestible compounds that, upon reaching the gut environment, selectively stimulate the growth and activity of probiotics. The ice cream that contains both probiotic and prebiotic components simultaneously is referred to as synbiotic or functional ice cream. In synbiotic ice cream, there is a synergistic effect between probiotics and prebiotics. When such ice cream is eaten and enters the large intestine, prebiotics are consumed by probiotics and enhance their population, leading to a decrease in the population of pathogenic bacteria. Ice cream has a good distribution capability for synbiotics among consumers. Studies have explored the possibility of adding each prebiotic to a special probiotic in ice cream. It seems that every probiotic microorganism needs special prebiotic compound to express better growth as well as survivability. *L. casei* and *Bifidobacterium bifidum* are commonly used with resistant starch in the production of synbiotic ice cream. Also, microencapsulation may be used as a novel method for directly protecting probiotics, preventing the adverse effects of ice cream and the gastrointestinal system, and increasing the synergistic effect of probiotics and prebiotics in synbiotic ice cream (Homayouni 2008).

Probiotic Ice Cream: Science and Technology, First Edition. Aziz Homayouni-Rad.

8.2 Design of Synbiotic Ice Cream

The development of synbiotic ice cream is a complex endeavor that demands a deep understanding of both probiotics and prebiotics. From a research and development perspective, creating functional synbiotic ice cream requires collaboration across various fields, including food technology, food biotechnology, nutrition, medicine, and food chemistry. The goal is to produce innovative products that can positively impact physiological parameters related to health and disease prevention. The design and development of functional synbiotic ice cream is a multifaceted and costly process. It involves the consideration of numerous factors, such as sensory appeal, physicochemical and microbial stability, pricing, and other inherent functional properties, all of which are essential for success in the market. Furthermore, it is crucial to align these products with consumer expectations regarding functional synbiotic ice cream. In general, the creation of synbiotic ice cream is a holistic endeavor that merges scientific expertise, consumer insights, and innovative product development to deliver not only tasty ice cream but also potential health benefits. This interdisciplinary approach is essential for meeting both market demands and consumer expectations (Homayouni 2008).

8.3 Synbiotic Ice Cream Characterization

Several studies examined the efficacy of combining prebiotics and probiotics in synbiotic ice cream. One such study compared prebiotic, probiotic, and synbiotic ice creams. The probiotic ice cream contained two *Lactobacillus* species (*L. rhamnosus* and *L. casei*), which were used separately in fruit or vanilla-flavored ice cream. Inulin replaced part of the stabilizer in the prebiotic ice cream, while the synbiotic ice cream included 3 or 6% inulin along with either of the probiotic strains. All ice cream variations effectively maintained probiotic functionality (Homayouni 2008).

8.4 Technology of Synbiotic Ice Cream Production

Synbiotic ice cream can be produced easily by adding suitable prebiotic compounds as well as suitable probiotic microorganisms into ice cream formulation (Figure 8.1). Studies have shown that the probiotics present in ice cream do not undergo significant changes during one year of frozen storage. Frozen yoghurt provides a stable environment for the survival

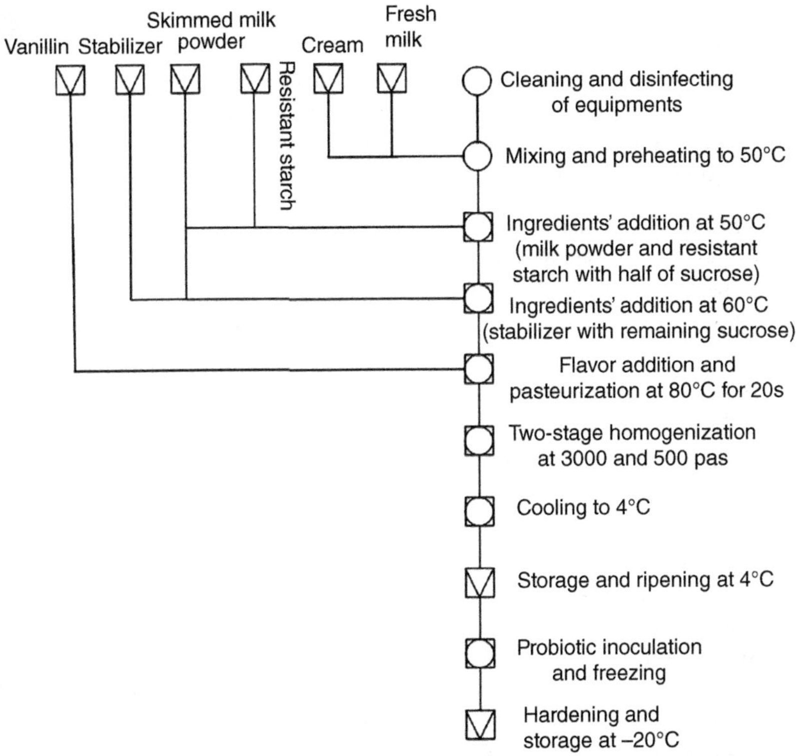

Figure 8.1 Symbiotic ice cream production process (Homayouni et al. 2008) / with permission of Elsevier.

and delivery of probiotics. Regular and fermented ice creams have good distribution capabilities among consumers. The low storage temperature of frozen dairy products provides ideal conditions for the long-term viability of probiotic bacteria. Fermented dairy desserts made from yoghurt have a low pH (around 4.5 or lower), which reduces the viability of live bacteria like *Lactobacillus acidophilus* and *Bifidobacterium* species due to the low pH. However, adding probiotic bacteria to ice cream does not pose a problem because the pH in ice cream (around 5.6–6.6) is ideal for their viability. The only challenge is air incorporation during freezing, which affects the viability of probiotics due to the presence of oxygen. The microencapsulation of probiotics in ice cream can prevent the toxic effects of oxygen on these bacteria. This approach can maintain their viability and effectiveness. The addition of prebiotics may increase the survivability of probiotics during refrigeration and storage (Homayouni et al. 2008). For the formulation of synbiotic ice cream, the following ingredients can be used: skim milk, heavy cream (40% fat), dry milk, sucrose, stabilizer, emulsifier, flavoring (vanillin), resistant starch, and probiotics. To produce synbiotic ice cream, the equipment to be used (a double-walled agitated tank as a formulation and pasteurization tank, and a homogenizer) is thoroughly cleaned and sanitized. Then, the ice cream ingredients, which have been preweighed, are mixed together in the following sequence:

1. Skim milk and heavy cream are added to the formulation tank and gently heated. When the temperature reaches 50°C, nonfat dry milk and resistant starch, mixed with half of the sucrose, are added slowly. The other half of the sucrose is mixed with stabilizer and emulsifier. Once the temperature reaches 60°C, this mixture is added to the formulation tank.
2. Heating continues until reaching 70°C, and the resulting mixture is kept at 70°C for 30 minutes to be pasteurized. During this time, while the agitator is active, flavoring agents are added.
3. The ice cream mixture is then subjected to a two-stage homogenization process in a homogenizer, first at 170 bar and then at 40 bar. The mixture is cooled to 4°C and held at this temperature for 12 hours to allow the mixture to mature.
4. Afterward, either free or microencapsulated probiotic cells are added to the nonfermented probiotic ice cream. Immediately after adding the probiotics, the mixture is frozen in a freezer with an expansion factor (overrun) of 100%, and then it is packaged in 100-gram cups and transferred to −20°C.

References

Homayouni, A. (2008). Effect of microencapsulation and resistant starch on the probiotic survival and sensory properties of synbiotic ice cream. PhD thesis. University of Tehran, Iran.

Homayouni, A. (2009). *Therapeutical Effects of Functional Probiotic, Prebiotic and Synbiotic Foods*. Tabriz, Iran: Tabriz University of Medical Sciences.

Homayouni, A., Azizi, A., Ehsani, M.R., and Yarmand, M.S. (2008). Effect of microencapsulation and resistant starch on the probiotic survival and sensory properties of synbiotic ice cream. *Food Chemistry* 111 (1): 50–55.

9

Postbiotic Ice Cream (Definition, Formulation, and Characterization)

9.1 Definition of Postbiotic Ice Cream

Postbiotic ice cream refers to ice cream containing alive probiotic cells and their metabolites that can be produced through either fermentation or nonfermentation methods, based on dairy or soy milk. Probiotics can be used in free form in ice cream formulations. After fermentation, the probiotic cells may be destroyed by ultrasound, heating, or other techniques, making the ice cream formula have health-promoting components when consumed in sufficient amounts. It is also possible to culture probiotic cells in culture media or whey and separate the cells by centrifugation and then rupturing the cells into postbiotics by ultrasound or heating. The obtained postbiotic may be added into nonfermented ice cream formulation immediately before freezing. Postbiotics are a category of biologically active compounds that are produced by the metabolic activity of probiotic microorganisms during the fermentation process. These compounds include various metabolites, cell wall components, enzymes, peptides, SCFAs, and other substances that have potential health benefits for the host. Ice cream has a good distribution capability for postbiotics among consumers. Studies have explored the possibility of adding postbiotics to both fermented and nonfermented ice cream. Among lactic acid bacteria, *Lactobacillus* and *Bifidobacterium* species are commonly used as suitable probiotics in the production of fermented dairy products. Postbiotics are resistant to the production and storage conditions as well as the harsh conditions of the digestive system making them a suitable alternative for substituting the live probiotic cells (Homayouni 2008; Homayouni, 2009).

Probiotic Ice Cream: Science and Technology, First Edition. Aziz Homayouni-Rad.

9.2 Postbiotics

The term “postbiotics” (also known as “nonbiotics”) encompasses all substances derived from probiotic microorganisms that are no longer viable, such as nonviable microbial cells, cell walls, lysates, fractions, secretions, components, and metabolites. When consumed in sufficient quantities as postbiotic supplements, these substances can present health benefits to the host, similar to the effects of live probiotic cells. Postbiotics possess specific chemical structures, exhibit a high safety profile, extended shelf life, and demonstrate strong stability in the presence of digestive enzymes, and the harsh conditions of the gastrointestinal tract. They have been observed to have no harmful effects on consumers. Additionally, substances produced by probiotic microorganisms, either secreted by live bacteria or released following bacterial breakdown (such as SCFAs, bacteriocins, enzymes, ethanol, diacetyl, peptides, hydrogen peroxide, teichoic acids, peptidoglycan-derived muropeptides, endo- and exo-polysaccharides, cell surface proteins, vitamins, plasmalogens, and organic acids) are also categorized as postbiotics. Probiotics offer a range of advantages, encompassing the alleviation of lactose intolerance, as well as immunomodulatory, hypocholesterolemic, anticarcinogenic, antidiarrheal, antidiabetic, and antihypertensive effects. Additionally, the provision of inactivated microbial cells (nonviable) or cell fractions, referred to as postbiotics, when administered in adequate quantities, can impart health benefits to individuals, similar to probiotics (Homayouni et al. 2020).

9.3 Design of Postbiotic Ice Cream

The development of postbiotic ice cream is a complex endeavor that demands a deep understanding of both the product itself and the preferences and needs of the consumers. It also necessitates effective management of customer knowledge. From a research and development perspective, creating functional postbiotic ice cream requires collaboration across various fields, including food technology, nutrition, medicine, and food chemistry. The goal is to produce innovative products that can positively impact physiological parameters related to health and disease prevention. The design and development of functional postbiotic ice cream is a multifaceted and costly process. It involves the consideration of numerous factors, such as sensory appeal, physicochemical and microbial stability, pricing, and other inherent functional properties, all of which are essential for success in the market. Furthermore, it is crucial to align these products with consumer expectations regarding functional postbiotic products. In general, the creation of postbiotic ice cream is a holistic endeavor that merges scientific expertise, consumer insights, and innovative product development to deliver not only a tasty product but also potential health benefits. This interdisciplinary approach is essential for meeting both market demands and consumer expectations (Homayouni 2008; Homayouni et al. 2023).

9.4 Postbiotic Ice Cream Characterization

Numerous investigations have been conducted to assess the suitability of ice cream as a vehicle for delivery of postbiotics. These studies primarily focused on evaluating the taste and sensory acceptability of these products and their ability to preserve the viability of bacteria. Several studies explored the use of postbiotics alone in ice cream to determine their effectiveness as a postbiotic carrier (Homayouni 2008).

9.5 Technology of Postbiotic Ice Cream Production

Postbiotic ice cream can be produced successfully because studies have shown that the postbiotics present in ice cream do not undergo significant changes during frozen storage (Figure 9.1). Frozen yoghurt provides a stable environment for the delivery of postbiotics. Regular and fermented ice creams have good distribution capabilities among consumers. However, adding postbiotics to ice cream does not pose a problem (Homayouni 2008). For the formulation of postbiotic ice cream, the following ingredients can be used: skim milk, heavy cream (40% fat), dry milk, sucrose, stabilizer, emulsifier, flavoring (vanillin), and postbiotics. To produce synbiotic ice cream, the equipment to be used (a double-walled agitated tank as a formulation and pasteurization tank, and a homogenizer) is thoroughly cleaned and sanitized. Then, the ice cream ingredients, which have been preweighed, are mixed together in the following sequence:

1. Skim milk and heavy cream are added to the formulation tank and gently heated. When the temperature reaches 50°C, nonfat dry milk, mixed with half of the sucrose, is added slowly. The other half of the sucrose is mixed with stabilizer and emulsifier. Once the temperature reaches 60°C, this mixture is added to the formulation tank.
2. Heating continues until reaching 70°C, and the resulting mixture is kept at 70°C for 30 minutes to be pasteurized. During this time, while the agitator is active, flavoring agents are added.

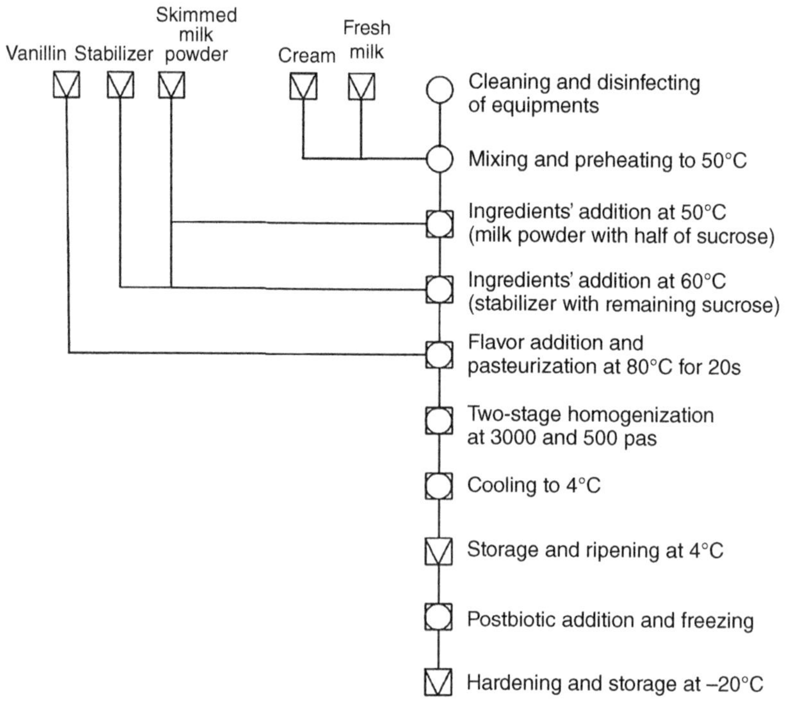

Figure 9.1 Postbiotic ice cream production process (Homayouni et al. 2008) / with permission of Elsevier.

3. The ice cream mixture is then subjected to a two-stage homogenization process in a homogenizer, first at 170 bar and then at 40 bar. The mixture is cooled to 4°C and held at this temperature for 12 hours to allow the mixture to mature.
4. Afterward, postbiotics are added to the nonfermented probiotic ice cream. Immediately after adding the postbiotics, the mixture is frozen in a freezer with an expansion factor (overrun) of 100%, and then it is packaged in 100-gram cups and transferred to −20°C.

References

Homayouni, A. (2008). Effect of microencapsulation and resistant starch on the probiotic survival and sensory properties of synbiotic ice cream. PhD thesis. University of Tehran, Iran.

Homayouni, A. (2009). *Therapeutical Effects of Functional Probiotic, Prebiotic and Synbiotic Foods*. Tabriz, Iran: Tabriz University of Medical Sciences.

Homayouni, A., Abbasi, A., Abedi, R., and Pouraga, B. (2023). Could postbiotics substitute probiotics. *Current Nutrition & Food Science* 19: 670–672.

Homayouni, A., Aghebati, L., Samadi, H. et al. (2020). Postbiotics as novel health-promoting ingredients in functional foods. *Health Promotion Perspectives* 10 (1): 3–4.

Homayouni, A., Azizi, A., Ehsani, M.R., and Yarmand, M.S. (2008). Effect of microencapsulation and resistant starch on the probiotic survival and sensory properties of synbiotic ice cream. *Food Chemistry* 111 (1): 50–55.

10

Functional Ice Cream (Ingredients and Processing)

10.1 Ice Cream Composition and Formulation

Ice cream is a frozen mixture composed of milk, sugar, fat, stabilizers, emulsifiers, flavoring agents, and color compounds. Within ice cream, three phases coexist: solid, liquid, and gas. Additionally, three systems: emulsion, suspension, and solution exist within ice cream. The composition of ice cream is highly complex, and it can be observed that there is a liquid system within the liquid phase (fat), a solid system within the liquid phase (casein suspension), and a gas system within the solid phase (air). Furthermore, various solutes are dissolved in the water present in ice cream (Figure 10.1). Therefore, ice cream is made up of the following components:

Milk fat in the range of 16–10%
Nonfat milk solids in the range of 12–9%
Sweeteners (sugar and glucose syrups) in the range of 16–12%
Stabilizers and emulsifiers in the range of 0.5–0.2%
Water (present in milk and other components) in the range of 64–55%

10.1.1 Total Solid Ingredients

In ice cream formulations, increasing the proportion of solid ingredients compared to water contributes to improved nutritional value, viscosity, texture, and overall structure of the product. The effects of increasing solid ingredients are more pronounced when incorporating carbohydrates, sweet cream, buttermilk solids, or egg yolks. Dry egg yolks, similar to dry buttermilk and sweet cream solids, enhance the air incorporation capacity of the mix and reduce freezing time. Increasing the amount of dry matter decreases the percentage of frozen water and increases the overrun, resulting in a minimum weight of 725.76 grams per gallon of ice cream. However, if the dry

Probiotic Ice Cream: Science and Technology, First Edition. Aziz Homayouni-Rad.

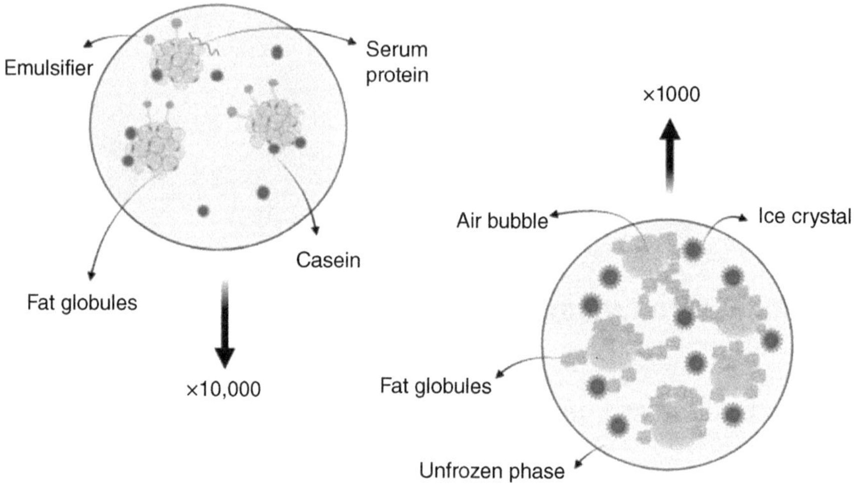

Figure 10.1 Schematic comparison of ice cream microstructure and initial mixture.

matter content exceeds 40–42%, the product can become wet and heavy. Additionally, excessive reduction of water content and addition of dry matter leads to a more yellowish color in the final product (Table 10.1).

10.1.2 Milk Fat

The best source of fat for ice cream formulation is sweet cream, which can enhance the ice cream's quality in terms of flavor. The importance of milk fat in ice cream formulation depends on the following factors:

1. Fat contributes to the richness of ice cream's flavor.
2. It softens the texture of the ice cream, leading to a smoother mouthfeel, especially when the ice cream is in contact with the roof of the mouth.
3. It improves the body of the ice cream, giving it a desirable structure.
4. It enhances the melting properties of ice cream.
5. It promotes smoother operation of the freezer due to the smoothness and fatty nature of the mixture during freezing.

However, excessive use of fat in ice cream formulation comes with the following limitations:

1. Increased costs.
2. Reduced aeration capacity (leading to delayed aeration).
3. Decreased consumer consumption due to concerns about excessive fat intake.
4. Elevated energy content of the ice cream.

Table 10.1 Advantages and limitations of using various types of ingredients in ice cream.

Raw material	Advantages	Limitations
Milk fat	Enhances desirable flavor, softens texture, mouth-coating richness, increases volume	High cost, slows air incorporation, high caloric content, potential health concerns
Nonfat solids	Improves texture, creates desired volume, increases overrun	Excessive amounts lead to crystallization, resulting in grittiness and cooked flavor
Sugar	Lowers freezing point, improves texture and flavor, reduces freezing temperature	Prolongs freezing time, excessive use reduces aeration capacity
Corn syrup solids	Low cost and sweetness, water-binding ability	Overuse can negatively impact flavor
Stabilizers	Softens texture, creates viscosity	Excessive use can make the product highly resistant to melting
Egg yolk solids	Enhances air incorporation capacity, imparts a custard-like flavor	Can curdle in a melted form
Total solids (TS)	Softens texture, increases nutritional content	Excessive reduction in coldness makes the product heavier, stickier, and wetter
Flavor enhancers	Improves acceptability	Undesirable sharpness and intensity of taste
Coloring agents	Enhances product appeal, aids in flavor identification	Some individuals may be sensitive to artificial colors

The milk fat plays a significant role in ice cream formulation. Fat enhances the desired flavor of ice cream and acts as a carrier for added flavors. Furthermore, it contributes to the desirable sensory qualities. Therefore, a balanced percentage of milk fat is used to achieve sensory attributes and comply with the set standards in ice cream formulation. Milk fat cannot decrease the freezing point of the mixture; instead, it reduces the rate of mixing the mixture. A high percentage of fat limits ice cream consumption, resulting in increased production costs. On the other hand, it increases the energy value of ice cream. Generally, a good ice cream contains around 12% fat content.

Fresh cream is the best source of milk fat. However, frozen cream, butter, yellow oil, and condensed milk can also be used. The importance of fat in forming the ice cream structure during the freezing stage is noteworthy. Fat increases the firmness of ice cream and its resistance to melting. Fat reduces the storage modulus. Excess fat leads to nonpliability and coarseness in texture. In cases of low-fat content, a soft, uniform, and relatively viscous texture is formed. Fat content and its type are used to classify various types of ice cream and frozen desserts based on the standards of different countries. Additionally, the use of vegetable fats is permitted in ice cream formulation as an alternative to milk fat. For producing good ice cream, it is essential to use fats with appropriate melting points. Fats with high melting points can create a waxy sensation in the mouth. Conversely, using fats with low melting points for making the foam is quite difficult. For this reason, it has been emphasized that dairy fat should have a suitable melting range to achieve a desirable creaminess and ideal dairy flavor in ice cream. In ice cream, palm oil and coconut oil can also be used due to their melting range being quite similar to dairy fat.

The most significant issue in ice cream is the oxidation of its fat. The melting range of milk fat triglycerides is quite broad, ranging from about −40 to +40°C. Thus, a combination of liquid and crystalline fat exists in fat globules at refrigeration temperature. The ratio of solid to liquid fat is highly important in the structure of ice cream, as partial encapsulation of fat globules requires crystalline fat. During the melting of ice crystals in ice cream, the accumulated fats help maintain the texture of the product to some extent. Sensory tests reveal that reducing fat content leads to excessive icy and crumbly texture degradation, accompanied by a decrease in the cream's aroma and taste, while the aroma and taste of dry milk intensify. Moreover, the number of air bubbles decreases.

10.1.3 Milk Solids-Non-fat (MSNF)

The main sources of milk solids-non-fat include:

1. Condensed skim milk
2. Milk powder (produced through spray drying and low-temperature methods).

Additionally, to source milk solids-non-fat, whole sweetened condensed milk, sweetened condensed skim milk, frozen and concentrated skim milk, buttermilk powder, concentrated buttermilk, full-cream condensed milk, concentrated whey, and whey powder can be used. Milk solids-non-fat or serum solids comprise lactose, caseins, whey proteins, salts, and ash.

The reasons for using milk solids-non-fat in ice cream formulation can be summarized in several points:

1. Improvement of ice cream texture due to functional properties of proteins.
2. Contribution to body formation and increased ice cream resistance against chewing.
3. Allowing greater aeration in the product without causing the texture to become icy or flaky.
4. Cost-effectiveness of these ingredients, especially in the case of whey powder.

The limitations of using excessive amounts of milk solids-non-fat in ice cream formulation include the development of an undesirable taste in the product and an increase in the lactose content in the formulation, which can lead to the issue of the texture becoming sandiness in the ice cream. Additionally, high levels of lactose can reduce the freezing point of the mix, resulting in delayed freezing of the product. Milk solids-non-fat, known as MSNF, include proteins, lactose, and mineral components of milk. The percentage composition of these components in MSNF is approximately 36.7% protein, 55.5% lactose, and 7.8% minerals. MSNF plays a crucial role in creating ice cream texture and body, influencing the product's storage properties. It is also a cost-effective ingredient with high nutritional value, though it does not contribute significantly to flavor. The lactose present complements the sweet taste created by other sugars. The salts in MSNF contribute to a mild salty taste in the ice cream, modifying the final product's flavor. Proteins lead to increased cohesion and softening of the ice cream, preventing the formation of a weak body and coarse texture. However, excessive amounts of MSNF can lead to excessive saltiness and a cooked taste in the ice cream, resulting in a soggy and sandy texture. In this case, the sandy texture is due to the high concentration of lactose. Determining the maximum amount of MSNF in ice cream is challenging. To calculate the maximum amount of serum solids in ice cream, the sum of all solid components except MSNF is subtracted from 100, and the result is divided by a factor ranging from 6.4 to 7.4. The choice of the factor depends on whether a rapid or slow freezing rate is desired. For a mix containing 12% fat, 15% sugar, and 0.3% stabilizers, the maximum MSNF for rapid freezing would be around 11.36%. As the amount of MSNF increases, viscosity and resistance to melting increase, while the freezing point decreases.

$$\frac{100 - (12 + 15 + 0.3)}{6.4} = \frac{72.7}{6.4} = 11.36$$

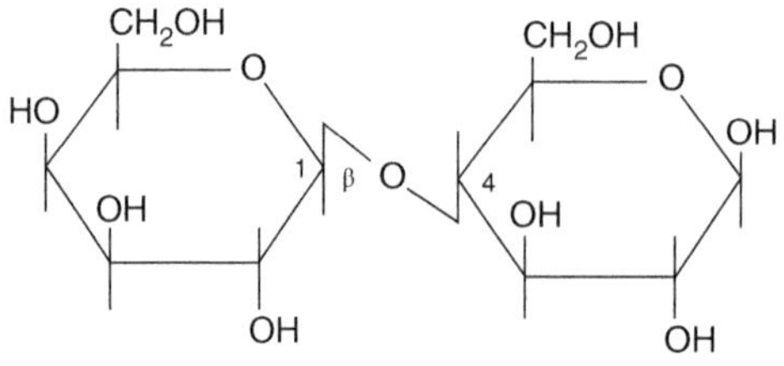

Figure 10.2 The structure of milk sugar (lactose).

10.1.4 Sweeteners

Consumers often prefer sweet ice cream, which is why it is logical to use 12–16% sweeteners in ice cream formulation. Sweeteners improve the texture and enhance the palatability of ice cream. Being the most cost-effective source of dry matter in ice cream, they also intensify the ice cream's flavor. Sugars like lactose found in milk lower (Figure 10.2) the freezing point of ice cream and increase the level of unfrozen water at ice cream consumption temperatures (from −15 to −18 °C). If unfrozen water is absent from the ice cream structure, its spoonability (scoopability) significantly decreases. Sweeteners prevent the total solids and sugar content of the product from increasing by more than 42 and 16%, respectively. Beyond these levels, the ice cream becomes excessively wet and sticky. Sweeteners in solution form cause a reduction in the freezing point of the mixture, leading to slower freezing and requiring lower temperatures for firming the product. Apart from their impact on ice cream quality, sweeteners, except those with low caloric or nutritional value, are considered the most inexpensive components of total solids in the mix.

Sucrose is the most important sweetener used in ice cream formulation. The reason for this is its ability to impart a very desirable taste to the product. Sucrose is a disaccharide composed of glucose and fructose. Nowadays, the substitution of corn syrups for all or part of the sucrose in ice cream has become a common practice. This not only provides economic benefits and sweetness but also contributes to the production of a soft, chewable texture and an increased shelf life for the ice cream. The ratio of these types of sweeteners, which are used in conjunction with sugar, depends on the following factors:

1. The level of dry matter in the ice cream mixture.
2. The desired percentage of sugar in the mixture.
3. The effects of these substances on the characteristics of the mixture, such as viscosity, freezing point, and aeration capability.
4. The concentration and potency of the above-mentioned sweetening agents.

Corn syrup, which serves as a substitute for sucrose, is a mixture of dextrose, maltotriose, and dextrose oligomers obtained through partial hydrolysis of starch by acid or enzymes. Its precise composition depends on the degree of hydrolysis, often represented as DE (dextrose equivalent). DE indicates the level of reducing sugars present as dextrose and is calculated as a percentage of its content in the total dry matter. Higher DE values can result in excessive molecular weight reduction. However, DE alone cannot determine the exact sugar composition, as various combinations of sugars can have the same DE value. Corn syrups generally possess less sweetness compared to sucrose. When carbohydrates react with hydrogen in the presence of a catalyst, sugar alcohols such as sorbitol are formed from dextrose, lactitol from lactose, and mannitol from mannose. The sweetness of these sugar alcohols is generally lower than sucrose, and they are not fully digested by the human body, resulting in only half of the caloric value of regular sugars. Therefore, these types of sugar alcohols are recommended for individuals with diabetes. Excessive consumption of these sugar alcohols can lead to diarrhea. The absence of sweeteners in ice cream formulation results in a bland product, while higher amounts of sugar can mask the desired flavor. Hence, a sugar content of around 14–16% in ice cream formulation is considered desirable. Sugars contribute to increased viscosity and dry matter of the mixture, improving the texture and body of the ice cream, provided the dry matter content does not exceed 40% and the sugar content does not exceed 16%. Beyond these limits, the ice cream tends to become too moist and sticky. Soluble sugars lower the freezing point of the mixture, reducing the freezing rate and requiring lower temperatures for firming up the ice cream.

10.1.5 Stabilizers

Stabilizers are a group of polysaccharides or protein compounds responsible for increasing the viscosity of the nonsolid portion of ice cream. They react with water molecules, rendering them immobile, and preventing their migration from one point to another within the ice cream. This process contributes to the softening and chewiness of the ice cream. If stabilizers are not used in ice cream formulation, the ice cream quickly becomes coarse, rough, and icy. This is due to the migration of free water and the growth of ice crystals within the ice cream. From a nutritional perspective, stabilizers are a suitable source of soluble fibers. Although they are derived from natural sources, they are classified as food additives according to European regulations and are therefore associated with an E-number (a specific number assigned by the European Union for food additives). The presence of hydroxyl groups in stabilizers allows them to form hydrogen bonds with

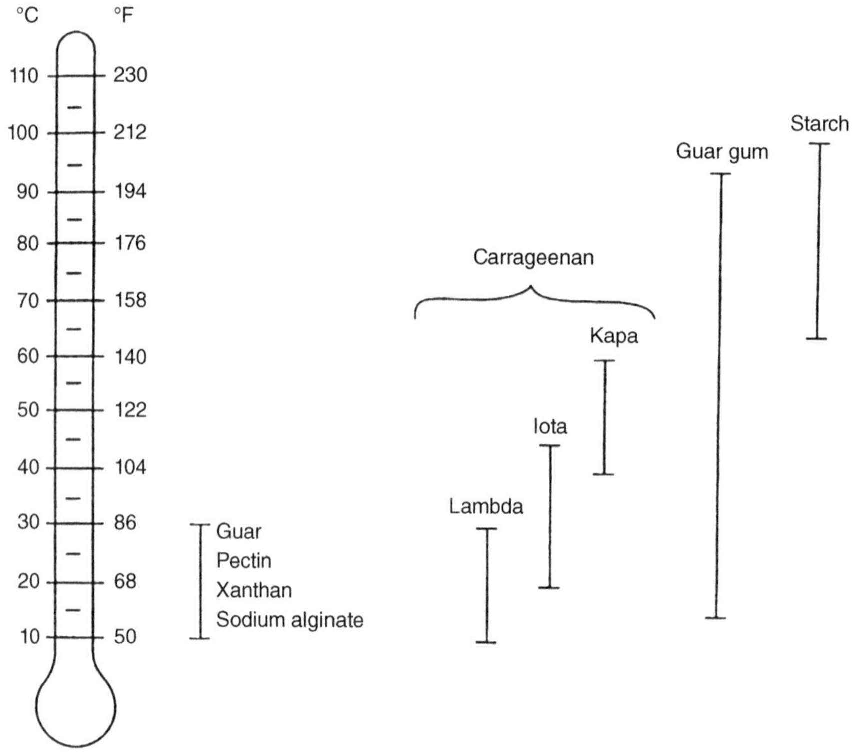

Figure 10.3 Solubility temperatures of some polysaccharide stabilizers.

water molecules. They typically consist of around 10^3 monomer units and have molecular weights ranging from 10^5 to 10^6. Because stabilizers have large molecules, they are not easily soluble in water. Some of them require higher temperatures or more vigorous stirring for hydration, and even at low concentrations, they can produce solutions with high viscosity. The dissolution temperature of some polysaccharide stabilizers is shown in Figure 10.3.

The smaller the ice crystals in ice cream, the harder it is to detect them when touching the ice cream with your tongue. Nowadays, during the transportation and distribution of ice cream, the possibility of the cold chain being broken exists. Ice cream may experience some melting in refrigerated trucks specially designed for transportation and in supermarkets. As the product is cooled again, the water refreezes. This process is referred to as heat shock. Each time this phenomenon occurs, the ice cream becomes more icy in texture. By using stabilizers, we can prevent this phenomenon (Figure 10.4).

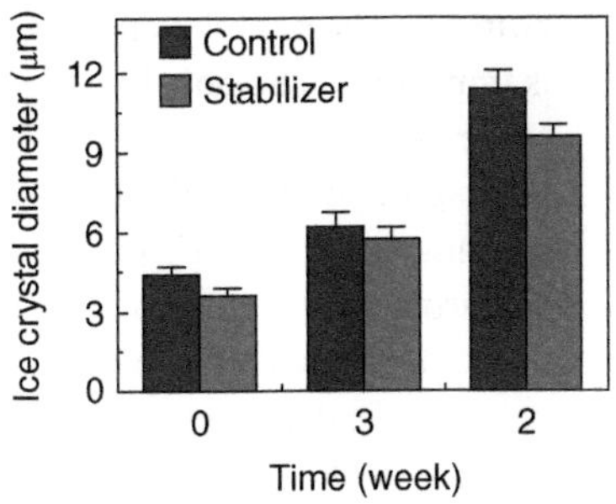

Figure 10.4 The effect of stabilizers on ice crystal size during ice cream storage.

The function of stabilizers in ice cream can be summarized as follows:

1. Creating a soft texture and body by increasing viscosity in the nonfrozen phase of ice cream.
2. Delaying or reducing the growth of ice crystals during storage.
3. Producing a uniform and melt-resistant product.
4. Assisting in the even distribution of flavoring agents in the ice cream.
5. Forming a stable base.
6. Generating a firm product suitable for cutting and packaging.
7. Preventing the formation of ice cream surface wrinkles.
8. Reducing the migration of water from the inside to the outside of the ice cream.

However, there are limitations to using stabilizers in ice cream, including:

A. Undesirable melting characteristics due to high viscosity.
B. High viscosity of the mixture before freezing, leading to difficulties in pumping and transferring the mixture in pipes and also within the freezer.
C. Creation of a heavy, wet, and gummy body.

Balancing the benefits of stabilizers with these potential drawbacks is a crucial consideration in ice cream formulation, as the goal is to achieve the desired texture and quality while avoiding negative effects on the product's overall characteristics. The stabilizers currently used in the ice cream industry include the following:

1. **Carob/Locust Bean Gum (LBG):**
   Locust bean gum contains 88% galactose and mannose, 5% various polysaccharides, 6% protein, and 1% ash. The main chain of this polysaccharide is composed of mannose, with galactoses attached as side branches. This gum is partially soluble in cold water and needs to be heated to temperatures above 85°C to be fully hydrated. Carob seed

gum is the best stabilizer for many ice creams, and its ability to form gels is important. The only limitation to its usage is its relatively high cost.

2. **Guar Gum:**
   Guar gum is derived from the endosperm of the guar plant, which belongs to the legume group. This type of gum has a structure similar to carob seed gum, consisting of a skeleton made up of mannose units, about half of which have galactose branches. The higher proportion of galactose units in this gum allows guar to be soluble in cold water as well. Guar gum creates high viscosity at low concentrations, but it undergoes degradation at high temperatures. Due to the neutral structure of guar, the viscosity it produces is much less affected by the pH of the environment. This gum is more cost-effective compared to carob seed gum.
3. **Carboxymethyl Cellulose (CMC):**
   This gum is also referred to as cellulose gum and easily dissolves in ice cream mixtures. It has a high water-holding capacity and on its own, it forms a weak gel. Additionally, it acts as an emulsifier and is used in ice cream products at a level of 0.1–0.2%. Its functional properties are suitable for both frozen dairy desserts and fruit-based ice creams. It also has a moderate cost.
4. **Xanthan Gum:**
   The main building blocks of xanthan gum include glucose, mannose, and galacturonic acid. Despite its high molecular weight, it easily dissolves in both cold and hot water. Even in small amounts, it forms highly viscous solutions and its viscosity is noticeably reduced upon agitation. Overall, changes in pH do not have a significant effect on the viscosity it creates. It is important to note that the use of xanthan gum in ice cream is not very common due to its high cost.
5. **Carrageenan:**
   Carrageenan is a complex polysaccharide composed of galactose and α-3,6-anhydrogalactose esters. It is made up of different polymer groups with distinct properties, including kappa, iota, and lambda carrageenans. Carrageenans are polyelectrolytes that, in aqueous solutions, form gels when heated and cooled in the presence of cations such as K^+ or $Ca^{2+.}$ Kappa carrageenan, in particular, plays a specific role in ice cream. Adding 0.02% of it can reduce the separation of milk protein and polysaccharides phases.
6. **Sodium Alginate:**
   Sodium alginate is a polysaccharide composed of glucuronic and mannuronic acid units, forming a negatively charged polymer chain that is linked to sodium ions through ionic bonds. Calcium ions or

other divalent cations can link to two different polymer molecules with negative charges, causing molecular interference and gel formation. In ice cream, alginate is mixed with phosphate, citrate, or tartrate ions to prevent premature gelling due to the calcium present in milk solids. The primary advantage of alginate is its resistance to acidic conditions, especially when exposed to heat. While other stabilizers lose their effectiveness under such conditions, alginate retains its properties.

7. **Gelatin:**
   Gelatin is a mixture of high-molecular-weight peptides derived from collagen and is typically used as a gelling agent or firming agent. It is commonly used to create gels. However, nowadays, other stabilizers are often used in place of gelatin.
8. **Tragacanth:**
   This gum is composed of two different polymers:
   1. Tragacanthin, which makes up 60 to 70% of the gum, is a polymer of D-galacturonic acid with side branches of galactose, L-fucose, and xylose.
   2. Bassorin, a polymer of methoxylated organic acids, makes up the remaining portion. Its main component is 75% L-arabinose. Unlike tragacanth, it is insoluble in water and forms a gel at around 0.5% concentration. An important characteristic of k-carrageenan is its stability against acidic environments and heat.
9. **Oat Gum:**
   Oat gum is a natural gel-forming substance derived from the seeds of the oat plant. It exhibits distinct chemical composition and physical properties. Oat gum is known for its role in delaying the measurement of blood glucose and sugar levels after meals, which could be beneficial for diabetes management. Additionally, it finds application in the production of food, cosmetic, pharmaceutical, and industrial products. This gum can serve as a food additive to provide gelling, thickening, and stability in various materials. It is also utilized as an additive in cosmetic and personal care products to enhance viscosity and shelf life.
10. **Pectin:**
    Pectin has a molecular structure composed of galacturonic acid molecules connected to each other through α-1,4 linkages. Other components such as arabinan, xylan, galactan, and rhamnose are attached to positions 2 and 3 of galacturonic acid. The presence of rhamnose causes the chain to form a helical structure. Pectin is a colloidal substance with a negative charge and is unstable at alkaline pH levels. It is sensitive to heat. The solubility of pectins increases with higher degrees of esterification and lower molecular weight. Pectins

are categorized into high-ester pectins with degrees of esterification above 50% and low-ester types with degrees of esterification below 50%. High-ester pectins are further divided into rapid-set and slow-set categories. Rapid-set pectins are esterified over 70% and form a gel at hot temperatures (around 80°C), with their gel strength directly related to molecular weight. Slow-set pectins have degrees of esterification ranging from 50 to 70%, and their gelling ability is dependent on the degree of esterification. Low-ester pectins have degrees of esterification below 50% and do not require sugar and acid for gelling; they only need divalent ions, particularly Ca^{2+} and Mg^{2+}. As previously mentioned, stabilizers are used to prevent the formation of large ice crystals in ice cream. These substances have high water-holding capacities and contribute to the softness of the final product's texture and body. In addition to inhibiting crystal growth during storage, stabilizers create uniformity in the product, increase resistance to melting, and enhance the creamy characteristics of ice cream. The effects of stabilizers on taste are indirect. They increase the viscosity of the mixture and reduce its air incorporation ability. Stabilizers do not impact the freezing point. The amount of stabilizer used depends on the type of stabilizer, the dry matter content of the mixture, the type of equipment, and other factors. Generally, stabilizers are used at a level of 0.2–0.3%. The most common stabilizers include sodium alginate, sodium carboxymethyl cellulose, guar gum, carob gum, carrageenan, gelatin, and pectin. When using alginate, there is no need for pasteurization. Carboxymethyl cellulose creates a thickened state in the product. Gelatin produces a thin mixture that requires aging. Pectin is used alone or in combination with gums to stabilize syrups and frozen desserts. Excessive stabilizer amounts lead to a heavy and wet body and increased resistance to melting.

10.1.6 Emulsifiers

Emulsifiers are substances that improve the structure of fats and the distribution of air within ice cream. They contribute to a softer texture and proper meltdown characteristics in the product. Because an emulsifier molecule has both hydrophilic (water-loving) and hydrophobic (fat-loving) parts, it positions itself at the interface of water and fat phases, reducing the surface tension between the two phases in the common phase (Figure 10.5). As a result, the surface tension of the emulsion's two phases is reduced. Ultimately, the ice cream's texture becomes softer, and its melting properties are enhanced.

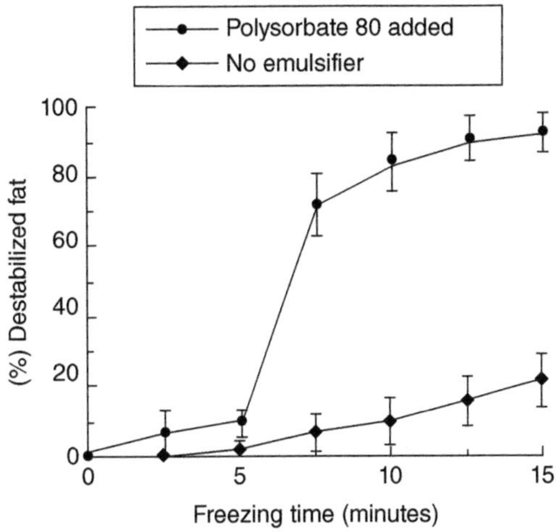

Figure 10.5 The impact of emulsifiers on fat globule destabilization in ice cream.

The first emulsifier used in ice cream was egg yolk, but nowadays, in ice cream formulation, both mono- and diglycerides and polysorbates are commonly employed as emulsifiers. Egg yolk is a mixture composed of approximately 50% water, 16% lecithin, 23% other fats, 0.3% carbohydrates, and 1.7% minerals. Lecithin contains phosphatides and phospholipids and is typically pasteurized, sugar-tempered, frozen, and spray-dried in ice cream factories. Normally, the solid egg yolk percentage in ice cream mix is around 0.5–3%. Higher levels of egg yolk are used in the production of premium ice creams to impart an egg-yolk flavor. Monoglycerides are esters of glycerol with a single fatty acid molecule, while diglycerides are esters of glycerol with two fatty acid molecules. Monoglycerides and diglycerides possess surface activity due to the hydrophobic fatty acid tail and the hydrophilic glycerol end. The properties of these molecules are determined by the fatty acids they contain. They are produced by hydrolyzing soybean oil and palm oil to a specific extent. Monoglycerides and diglycerides usually contain 40–60% monoglycerides along with diglycerides and a small amount of triglycerides. Saturated types are commonly used in ice creams, containing mostly stearic and palmitic acids (like glycerol monostearate), making up around 0.3% of the ice cream mixture. Mono- and diglycerides are derived from the partial hydrolysis of fats and plant and animal oils. Polysorbate 80, which is a sorbitan ester, consists of a sorbitol molecule linked to oleic acid, with added ethylene oxide groups for improved water solubility. Other sources of emulsifiers include buttermilk and glycerol esters, all of which are composed of fats and carbohydrates and play crucial roles in the composition of many foods. Emulsifiers and stabilizers collectively make up less than 0.5% of the weight of the ice cream formulation and have been recognized

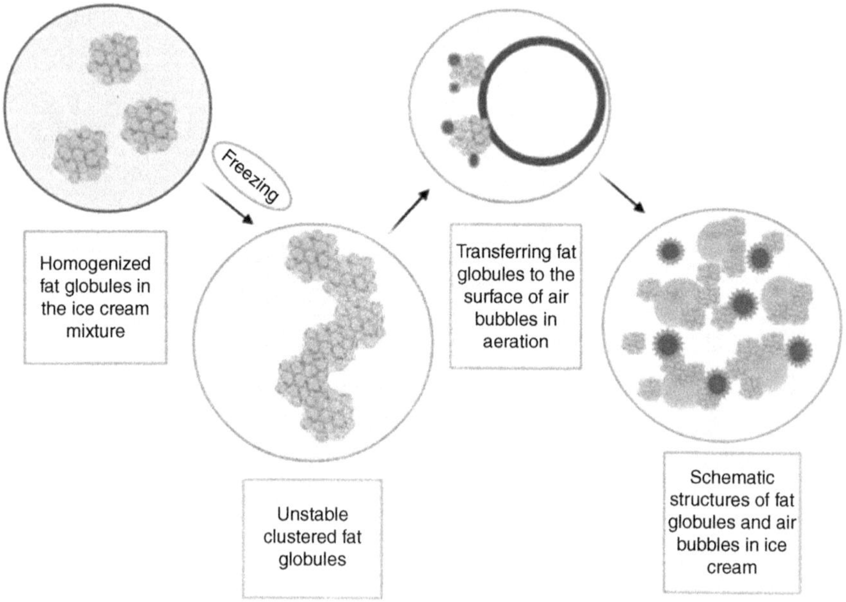

Figure 10.6 Relative destabilization of lipid droplets and formation of three-dimensional structures in ice cream.

as GRAS in terms of food safety and hygiene. Emulsifiers interact with the surface of fat globules, causing them to become unstable. As a result, the fat globules experience partial coalescence and merge with air bubbles, forming an extensive network and three-dimensional structure. This process leads to a softer ice cream texture and a slower melting rate (Figure 10.6).

Emulsifiers are used to produce a product with a soft texture and body that possesses drying properties, enhancing the ability of the mix to incorporate air. Emulsifiers extensively employed in ice cream production include monoacylglycerides, diacylglycerides, sorbitan esters, and polyoxyethylene sorbitan esters (polysorbates). These compounds are utilized in ice cream mixtures at levels ranging from 0.1 to 0.4%. Egg yolk is also employed as an emulsifier. Excessive amounts of emulsifiers can delay the melting of ice cream, resulting in subpar texture and body.

10.1.7 Flavors and Colors

Flavor is typically considered the most important characteristic of ice cream. The type of flavoring substance used in ice cream is influenced by the quality of the ice cream mixture. If the mixture contains a negligible amount of improper flavor, it can overshadow the added flavor. Furthermore, the type and intensity of flavor used depend on consumer demand. Both natural and synthetic flavorings can be utilized in ice cream. Vanilla is often used to flavor ice cream, with its synthetic version called vanillin (Figure 10.7). On the other hand, ice cream should have an appealing color that is closely associated with its flavor. Colors are often chemically derived and are available in both liquid and powdered forms on the market. Ice cream manufacturers often prefer powdered colors for economic reasons.

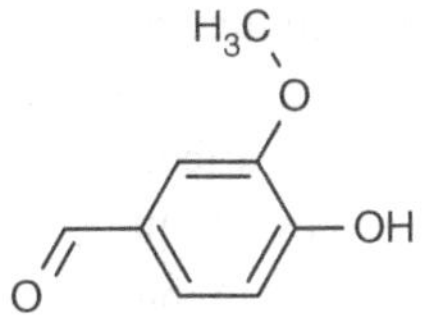

Figure 10.7 Chemical structure of vanillin.

10.1.8 Water Content and Gases in Ice Cream

Ice cream is a physicochemical system in which the gaseous phase (air) is dispersed in the liquid phase (water) or in the solid phase, or in a mixture of solid and liquid phases. Therefore, the continuous phase includes an emulsion, where a portion of it is frozen, and in the unfrozen portion, ice crystals and frozen fat globules are encapsulated. The water present in the ice cream mixture is primarily sourced from liquid dairy products or added water in the formulation. The amount of air in ice cream is also of significant importance, as it affects the product's quality, profitability, and conformity to standards. To achieve better quality, it is necessary to incorporate an appropriate amount of air uniformly into the ice cream. Recent studies have investigated the injection of gases other than air into the ice cream mixture. The results of these studies indicate that adding very fine solid CO_2 particles during the ice cream production process yields a highly interesting and acceptable product.

10.1.9 Optional Ingredients and Components in Ice Cream Formulation

Several specific compounds are used for their desirable effects in preparing ice cream mix and the final product. In cases where aromatic and flavorful materials are used in the production of frozen pastry and nut-based ice cream, salt can be employed, with a 0.1% salt content being sufficient. Caseinat derivatives, especially sodium caseinates, increase aeration and volume of the product. They can stabilize an emulsion that might not be stable during freezing due to low-fat content. In such cases, the product's texture will not be dry and firm. Mineral salts accompanied by citrates, phosphates, calcium salts, and magnesium salts have an impact on the final product's quality and ice cream mix. Mineral salts are used in small quantities and affect attributes related to product transportation and appearance. Citrates and phosphates are suitable solvents for casein and enhance water absorption. Salts play a crucial role in creating stability in the ice cream mixture during the heating phase. Calcium salts reduce protein stability but provide a creamy appearance and pleasant color to the mixture and the final product. Small amounts of calcium sulfate influence the dryness and firmness of the frozen product, making it easier to release from the freezer. Solid materials low in lactose from milk containing proteins and mineral salts contribute to increased nutritional value and specific properties. They enhance the typical attributes and increase the amount of dry matter.

10.2 Stages of Ice Cream Production

The process of ice cream production consists of two main stages: mix preparation and freezing. Mix preparation involves blending and homogenizing the raw materials, homogenization, pasteurization, cooling, and aging. The necessary heat for pasteurizing the mixture is typically provided using steam. Boiler systems, such as fire-in-tube boilers, are commonly employed in food industries to generate steam. Therefore, the sequence of processes for ice cream production is as follows: mix preparation, pasteurization, homogenization, cooling, aging, addition of flavor and color ingredients, freezing, packaging, hardening, storage, loading of finished products, and equipment cleaning. The process flow and stages of ice cream production are illustrated in Figures 10.8 and 10.9.

10.2.1 Mix Calculations

The most important task in mix calculations involves determining the values of each component of the mixture based on the formula and the quantity of the final mixture. The formulas express the percentages of each ice cream component – fat, milk solids – nonfat, sugar, nonfat solids of syrup, stabilizer, and emulsifier. The sources for each ice cream component are chosen based on availability, quality, and cost. Below, the ice cream components and their sourcing are outlined.

1. Milk fat is sourced through cream and butter. Cream introduces MSNF and water into the mixture, in addition to milk fat. Butter also contains water and MSNF, aside from milk fat.

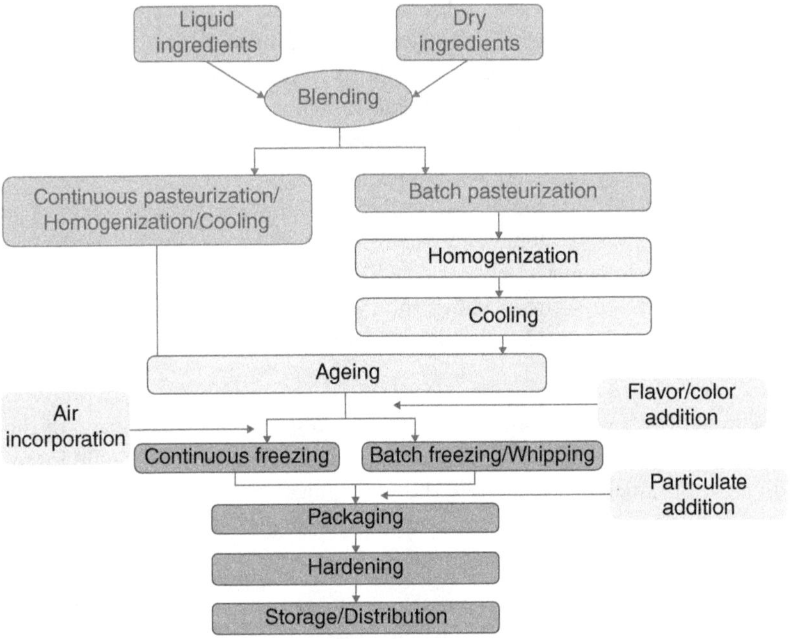

Figure 10.8 Ice cream production process.

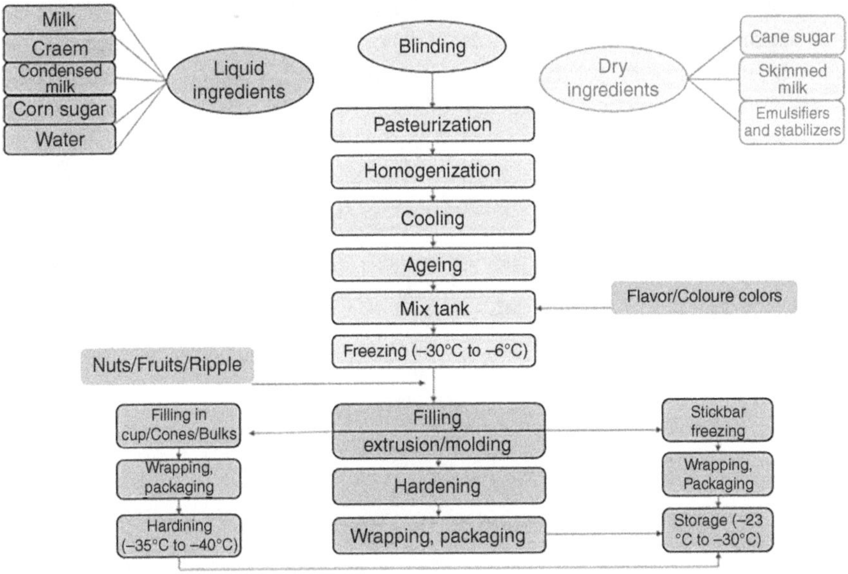

Figure 10.9 Stages of ice cream production.

2. Nonfat solids of milk are sourced from the following sources:
   Skim milk powder (which contains around 3% water).
   Nonfat condensed milk (which contains some water).
   Condensed milk (containing fat and water).
   Sweetened condensed milk (which contains water and sugar).
   Whey powder (which contains some water).
3. Water is sourced through skim milk, milk, and water itself. Skim milk also carries MSNF along with water. Whole milk contains fat and MSNF in addition to water.
4. Sweeteners are sourced using solid or liquid sugar and corn syrups. Liquid sugar is sucrose dissolved in water and introduces some water into the mixture.

The first step in mix calculations is selecting the sources for each of the mixture's components. If only one source is available for a specific ingredient, it is sufficient to multiply the percentage of that component by the required amount of the mixture. For example, to prepare 100 kilograms of a mixture with 10% sugar, you will have:

$$100(\text{kg Mix}) \times 10/100(\text{Sugar}) = 10\,\text{kg Sugar}$$

Therefore, the required amount of sugar will be 10 kilograms. If two different sources exist for a single component, we use the algebraic method of Al-Xarazmi (Pearson's) Square (Figure 10.10). For example, when you want to create a mixture with 20% fat, with fat sourced from two ingredients, skim milk (0% fat) and cream (35% fat), the Pearson's Square calculation will simplify the process. To solve the problem using Pearson's Square, start by writing the desired percentage of fat for the mixture (20) in the center of

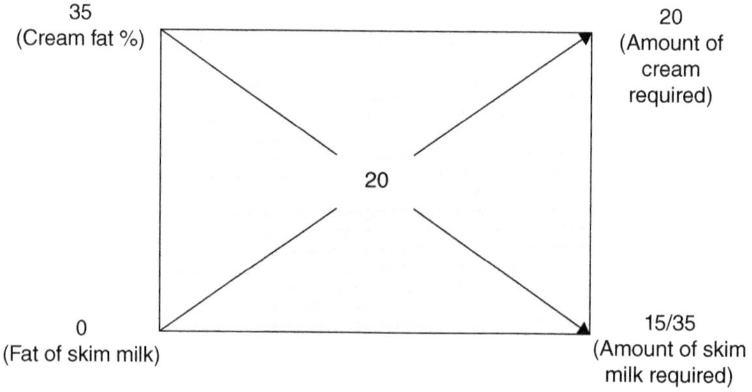

Figure 10.10 Ice cream mixture calculations using Xarazmi's (Pearson's) Square.

the square, then write the fat sources in the top-right corners of the square. In the next step, subtract the numbers located on each diagonal from each other and enter the result at the empty end of the same diagonal. This number indicates the required amount of the initial ingredient situated along that side of the square. In this example, the result of subtracting 20 from 35 is 15, which is written at the empty end of the corresponding diagonal and represents the 15 kilograms of skim milk required. Similarly, the result of subtracting 0 from 20 is 20, which is written at the empty end of the corresponding diagonal and indicates that 20 kilograms of cream are needed to create the required 35 kilograms of mixture ($20 + 15 = 35$).

One of the methods for mixture calculations involves using computer programs, which solve the mixture equations based on the principle of mass conservation and determine the quantity of each component. Manual calculations of the mixture can also be done using the serum point method, which will be explained in detail below. In this method, in order to create a standard and constant mixture, the percentages of components for each material used must be accurately estimated. Some ingredients used in the mixture have a constant amount of dry matter. Calculations based on dry matter are straightforward. In other cases, the percentages of each component present in the raw materials must be determined through chemical analysis. Information about raw materials has been provided.

A. Skim milk is a material whose composition can be determined through chemical analysis. Generally, the content of serum solids in skim milk is considered to be 9%. The fat content in skim milk is around 0.1–0.01%, which is usually neglected.
B. Nonfat dry solids include nonfat dry milk, whey powder, concentrated whey protein, and dry milk, which typically have 97% dry matter.
C. Cream's fat content is determined using the Babcock method or other approved methods. The percentage of nonfat solids in cream is calculated using the following formula, assuming that the nonfat solids content of skim milk is 9%:

$$0.09 \times (\text{Fat Percentage} - 100) = \text{Percentage of Serum Solids}$$

D. Milk, with its fat content determined using the Babcock method, and the percentage of its solid matter is obtained from the formula mentioned above.
E. Condensed milk's composition is determined through chemical analysis.
F. Sweeteners:
   1. Solid sugar, which is 100% solid matter.
   2. Liquid sucrose, which consists of 66% solid matter.

   3. Powdered dextrose glucose, which is 100% solid matter.
   4. Corn syrup powder, which is 100% solid matter.
   5. Corn syrup, which contains 80% solid matter.
   6. Liquid glucose, which contains 80% solid matter.
   7. Honey, which contains 80% solid matter.

G. Stabilizers and emulsifiers in powder form: Due to their small quantities in the mixture formulation, they consider these ingredients to be 100% solid matter.

H. Egg and egg products:
   1. Fresh whole egg, which contains 10% fat and 25% dry matter.
   2. Fresh and frozen egg yolks, which contain 33% fat and 50% solid matter.
   3. Egg yolk powder, which is 100% solid matter and constitutes 60% fat.

Example

The formulation of a sample ice cream is as follows:

Fat = 14%
Serum solids = 10%
Sugar = 15%
Emulsifier and stabilizer = 0.4%

To prepare 100 kilograms of the mentioned ice cream mixture, how much 80% fat butter, nonfat dry milk with 97% solids, water, sugar, and solid emulsifier and stabilizer are required?

Solution

1. First, let us calculate the amount of butter needed to achieve 14% fat in 100 kilograms of the mixture:
   Amount of mixture = 100 kg
   Desired fat percentage = 14%
   Amount of fat needed = Desired fat percentage × Amount of mixture
   Amount of fat needed = 14% × 100 = 14 kg
   Next, let us calculate the amount of nonfat dry milk needed to contribute to the serum solids content:
   Serum solids percentage = 10%
   Amount of mixture = 100 kg
   Amount of nonfat dry milk needed = Serum solids percentage × Amount of mixture
   Amount of nonfat dry milk needed = 10% × 100 = 10 kg
   The other ingredients, like water, sugar, and solid emulsifier and stabilizer, do not require any calculations since they are provided directly.
   14 kg fat × 100 kg butter/80 kg fat = 17.5 kg butter

2. Then, we will calculate the amount of nonfat dry milk needed to provide 10 kilograms of serum solids in 100 kilograms of the mixture. For this purpose, we will determine the amount of serum solids present in 17.5 kilograms of butter. It is known that 80% of butter constitutes fat, and the remaining 20% consists of skim milk. Within this 20%, 9% is MSNF (milk solids nonfat).
   Butter MSNF = 9 × 20% = 1.8%
   17.5 kg butter × 1.8 kg MSNF/100 kg butter = 0.315 kg butter MSNF
   Based on the calculations above, the nonfat dry milk should contain approximately 9.685 kilograms of solid matter. In other words:
   10 kg MSNF – 0.315 kg MSNF = 9.685 kg MSNF
   9.685 kg MSNF × 100 kg milk powder/97 kg MSNF = 9.98 kg milk powder
3. The required amount of sugar will be equal to:
   15/100 sugar × 100 kg mix = 15 kg sugar
4. Similarly, the required amount of emulsifier and stabilizer will be 0.4 kilograms per 100 kilograms of the mixture.
5. The required amount of water is equal to 100 minus the sum of the kilograms of the other components of the mixture:
   100 – (17.5 + 9.98 + 15 + 0.4) = 57.12 kg water
   Finally, to ensure the accuracy of the calculations, the sum of the weights of the mixture components should be equal to the desired amount of the mixture.

10.2.2 Preparing Ice Cream Mixture

The first step in ice cream production is preparing the mixture. Initially, the liquid ingredients are mixed together, and then the temperature is lowered to 55–65°C. In this stage, solid ingredients are added, and the mixture is vigorously mixed for about 10 minutes using powerful mixers to achieve uniform consistency (Figure 10.11). The mixing process is designed to efficiently blend, disperse, and dissolve the raw materials in minimal time and with optimal energy consumption. To achieve the best quality and proper utilization of raw materials, precise weighing of these materials is automated, and other materials with lower consumption are weighed separately and added manually. The mixing tank, along with the mixers, includes a means for heating the mixture, and insulation is applied to minimize heat loss. Liquid raw materials such as water, milk, and cream are weighed and then heated. Subsequently, the mixing process begins. Solid fats are melted before adding them to the mixture. Then, dry ingredients like sugar, stabilizers, and nonfat dry milk are added. Since dissolving stabilizers can be more challenging than other ingredients,

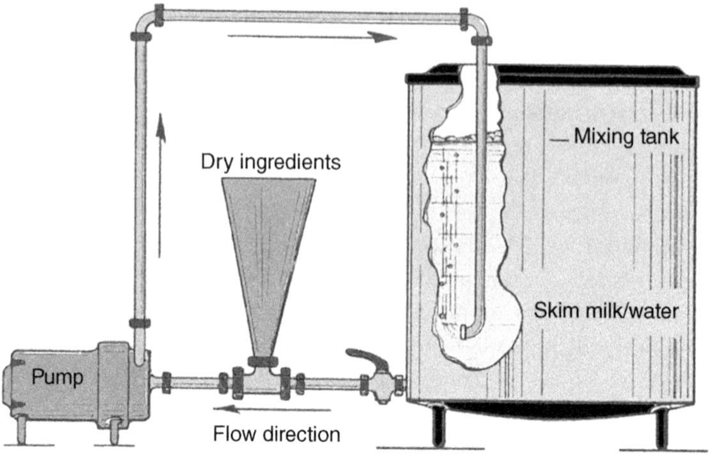

Figure 10.11 Mixing system for ice cream mix preparation.

they are mixed with a small amount of sugar (at least their own weight) before being added to the mixture to facilitate dissolution. Gradually, they are added to the tank and gently mixed to ensure uniform distribution in the mixture and prevent the formation of clumps due to incomplete dissolution of stabilizers. Nonfat dry milk and whey powder are also added gradually to prevent lump formation. The output from the tank passes through a strainer to separate any formed clumps from each other. Dairy products, especially proteins, are denatured at higher temperatures. For this reason, when such materials are added to the mixture, the mixture's temperature should not exceed 85°C. Colors and flavorings are also added at this stage, but if they are heat-sensitive, they should be added after pasteurization.

10.2.3 Homogenization

Homogenization of the ice cream mixture is achieved using a homogenizer device (Figure 10.12). The purpose of homogenization is to create a suspension in which the size of fat globules is reduced. Ideally, the diameter of fat globules should be less than two microns. As a result, in such a suspension, fat does not rise to the top, and no layer of cream is formed. Other advantages of homogenization include producing uniform ice cream with a smooth texture, improved air incorporation ability, reduced freezing time, prevention of butterfat crystallization in the freezer, and decreased stabilizer consumption. Homogenization is particularly necessary when using frozen cream, butter, yellow fat, or vegetable oils in ice cream formulation.

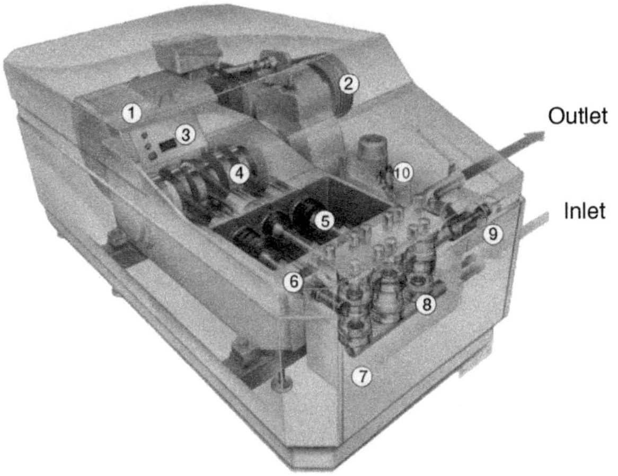

Figure 10.12 Homogenizer device 1: Main Motor, 2: Power Transmission Belt, 3: Pressure Gauge, 4: Plunger Rod, 5: Piston, 6: Piston Seal Cartridge, 7: Blocker, 8: Valves, 9: Homogenizing Head, 10: Hydraulic Pressure System. Source: Dr. ThienNonglam.

Homogenization of the ice cream mixture is performed based on the composition of the mixture and the shape of the valve at a pressure range of 2000–3000 PSI. This process is typically carried out in two stages as shown in Figures 10.13, 10.14, and 10.15. However, in formulations with fat content

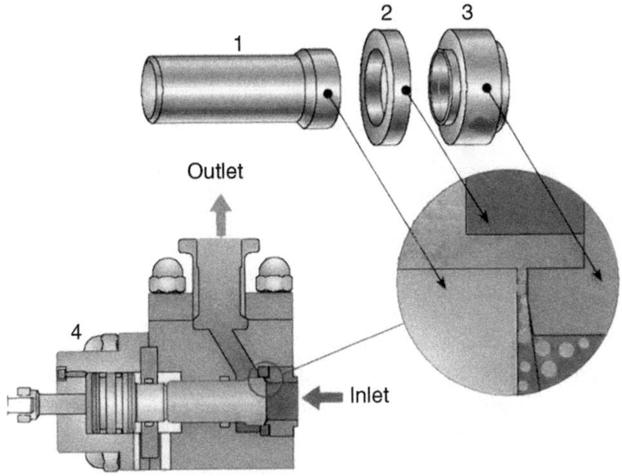

Figure 10.13 The components of a single-stage homogenizer: 1: Pressure component, 2: Connecting ring, 3: Head, 4: Hydraulic system.

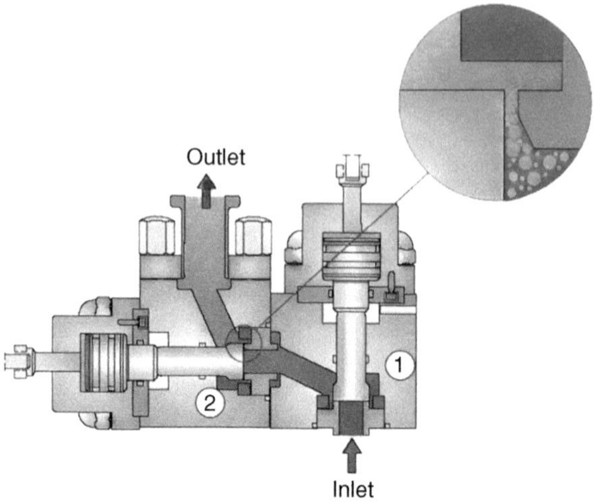

Figure 10.14 The components of a two-stage homogenizer: 1: First-stage head and 2: Second-stage head.

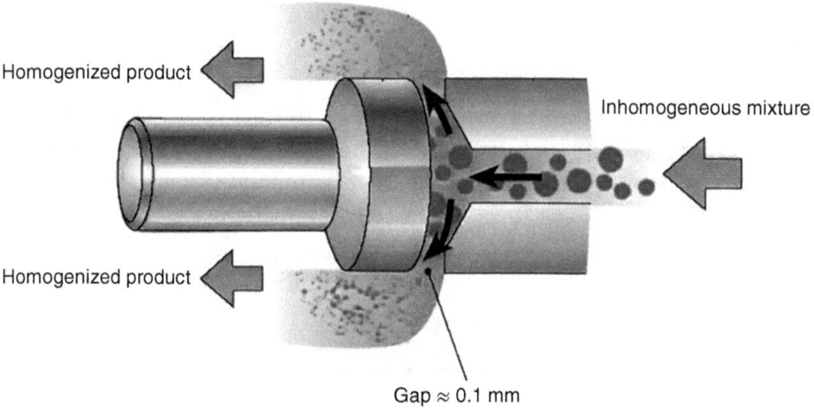

Figure 10.15 The mechanism of ice cream mixture homogenization.

less than 10%, a two-stage homogenization is not necessary. At higher pressures (5000–4000 PSI), the viscosity of the mixture decreases. The minimum pressure used in the homogenizer to achieve a stable product is 1450 PSI. The suitable temperature for homogenizing the mixture is around 63–76°C.

To bring the temperature of the mixture to the pasteurization temperature, a significant amount of energy is required. To increase energy efficiency, heating is done in two stages. In the first stage, the mixture is taken from the mixing tank and passes through a plate heat exchanger. This equipment is designed in a way that facilitates efficient heat transfer and easy cleaning, with two separate paths for the flow of the mixture. The first path is for the incoming mixture, and the second path is for the pasteurized and homogenized mixture. As a result, the incoming mixture undergoes heating, and the pasteurized and homogenized mixture goes through the first cooling stage, which should precede the next production step. In the second heating stage, the mixture is subjected to higher heat, which is provided by hot water in another section of the plate heat exchanger. At the end of this stage, the mixture's temperature must be such that, after homogenization, its temperature reaches the necessary level for pasteurization. It should be noted that to prevent undesirable flavors and denaturation, the temperature should not exceed 85°C. Table 10.2 presents the necessary pressures for single-stage and two-stage homogenizers (Tetra Pak Processing Systems AB, 1995).

During homogenization, the surface area of fat globules significantly increases. This results in insufficient membrane material to cover the newly formed globules. Additionally, the formation of a new membrane around the fat globule takes time. Therefore, mixtures with higher fat content should be homogenized at lower pressures. Otherwise, due to the closer proximity of fat globules in the fatty mixture, they tend to agglomerate and cluster together (Figure 10.16). Furthermore, in mixtures where butter, cream, plastic fats, etc., are used as the sole fat source, and concentrated dairy products are used as the sole source of MSNF, homogenization should be performed at lower pressures. Following homogenization, milk proteins adsorb onto the free surface of fat globules. The hydrophilic part of proteins usually gets absorbed toward the aqueous side of the fat–matrix interface, while the hydrophobic part is positioned toward the fat phase. Free casein, casein micelles, and soluble proteins possess different surface-active properties, leading to varying degrees of absorption by fat globules. For instance, casein absorption from soluble proteins is more prominent. Proteins are highly suitable for stabilizing fat-in-water emulsions and preventing fat globule coalescence. This is due to the formation of a tight and thick membrane around the fat globule, and the interaction between proteins on

Table 10.2 Homogenization pressure for mixtures with different fat percentages.

Fat percentage	Single-stage (kg/cm^2)	Two-stage – first head (kg/cm^2)	Two-stage – second head (kg/cm^2)
8	210	210	50
10	180	180	45
12	130	130	35
14	105	105	35
16	85	85	35

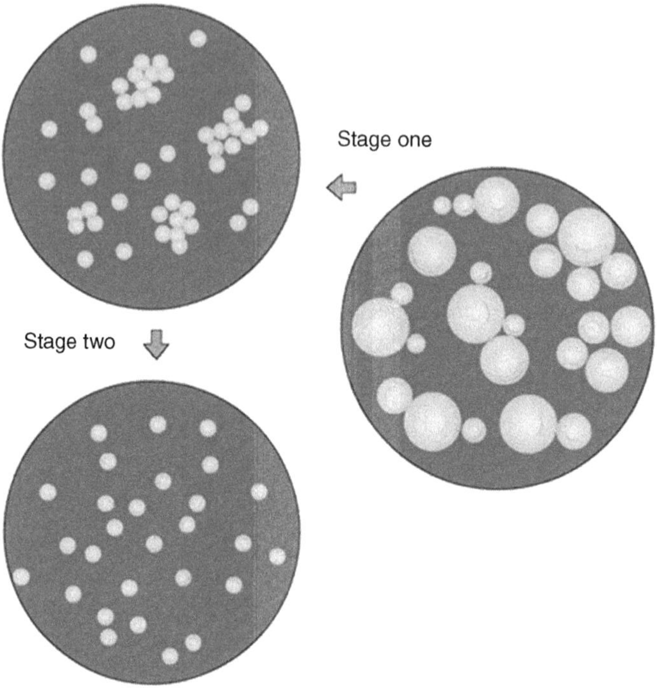

Figure 10.16 Microscopic scheme of milk fat globules during homogenization.

the outer surface of globules hinders their close approach, a phenomenon referred to as "steric stabilization." In other words, fat particles, because of the repulsion forces created by proteins enveloping them, do not come close to each other and remain stably suspended in the emulsion. Schematic distribution of fat globules around air bubbles in ice cream after freezing was shown in Figure 10.17.

10.2.4 Pasteurization

Pasteurization of the ice cream mixture is carried out to eliminate pathogenic microorganisms. On the other hand, raising the temperature facilitates the homogenization of the mixture and rapid disruption of fat globules. Pasteurizing the ice cream mixture involves rapidly increasing the temperature to a certain level, holding it at that temperature for a specified period, and then rapidly cooling the mixture to below 5°C. This process can be conducted in both continuous (Figures 10.18 and 10.19) and batch.

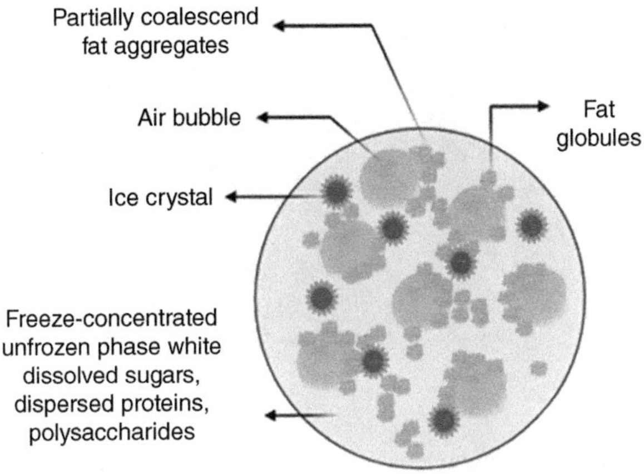

Figure 10.17 Schematic distribution of fat globules around air bubbles in ice cream after freezing.

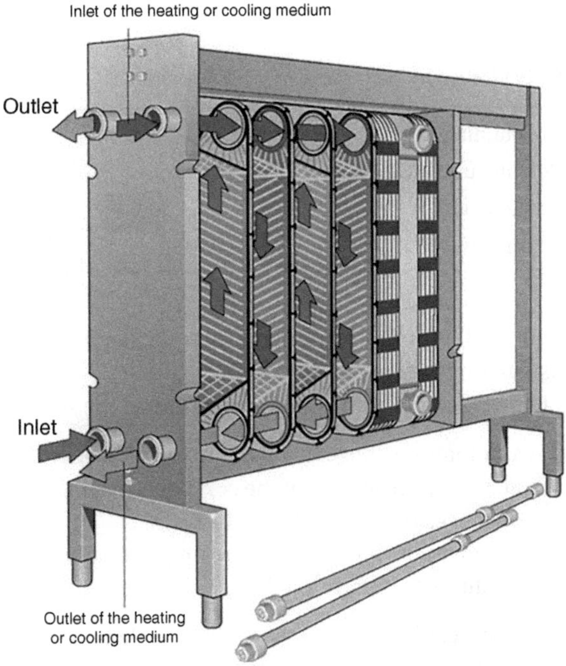

Figure 10.18 Continuous pasteurizer pages and the flow of the heat exchanger, chiller, and product.

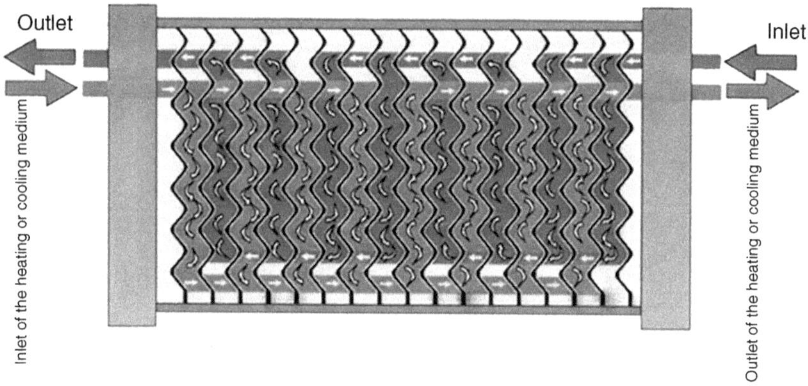

Figure 10.19 Continuous pasteurizer plates and the flow of the heat exchanger, chiller, and product.

Table 10.3 Time-temperature combinations for pasteurization of ice cream mixtures.

Pasteurization process type	Temperature (°C)	Time
Discontinuous (LTLT)	68	Minimum 30 minutes
Continuous (HTST)	79	Minimum 25 seconds
Continuous	90	3–1 seconds
Continuous	149–135	2–1 seconds

Table 10.3 provides the appropriate temperature-time combinations for pasteurizing the ice cream mixture.

The effects of pasteurization on ice cream mixture are as follows:

1. It eliminates pathogenic microorganisms from the mixture.
2. It aids in better mixing of the components.
3. It enhances the flavor of the ice cream.
4. It improves the quality of ice cream preservation.
5. It produces a uniform product.

The ice cream mixture is rapidly cooled to a temperature of 0–5°C immediately after homogenization and then stored in holding tanks. If the cooling process from 30 to 40°C down to below 5°C is done gradually, it increases the viscosity further and leads to slower melting of the resulting ice cream. Additionally, a lower temperature below 5°C prevents bacterial growth. Cooling the mixture to a temperature of 0–2°C enhances the freezing capacity.

10.2.5 Aging of Mix

The aging process is a crucial stage in ice cream production. Once the mixture is cooled, it is pumped into a tanker. The equipment along this path is designed in a way that minimizes the exposure of the mixture to atmospheric air or other sources of contamination. The mixture is maintained at a temperature between 0 and 4°C and is intermittently agitated. However, the agitation must be controlled to prevent the mixture from heating up. Heat-sensitive ingredients like colors, flavorings, and fruit pulps are typically added to the mixture at this stage. All the ingredients added after pasteurization must be microbiologically safe to avoid contaminating the pasteurized mixture. The changes that occur during the mixing phase include:

1. Crystallization of fat globules and enhanced adsorption of emulsifiers on the fat globule surfaces.
2. Stabilizers, especially gelatin, swell due to water absorption.
3. Milk proteins absorb water, and in the presence of emulsifiers, protein displacement from the fat globule membrane occurs. The rearrangement of the fat globule membrane occurs in a way that, as the mixture cools down, the surface activity of emulsifiers increases. This leads to the removal of proteins from the fat globule membrane. The result of all these reactions contributes to an increase in viscosity during the mixing conveyance phase.

Furthermore, during the mixing conveyance phase, the ability of the mix to incorporate air increases, resulting in a softer texture and body of the ice cream. It also enhances resistance to melting. Studies indicate that in industrial conditions, a duration of 4–3 hours for the mixing conveyance phase is sufficient for continuous freezers. However, for batch freezers, the mixing time should be longer. Especially for mixtures with high-fat percentages that are homogenized under low pressure, a 24-hour mixing period is required for desirable results. The temperature of the mixture during the mixing conveyance phase should not exceed 5°C. Below 5°C, the bacterial count does not increase.

10.2.6 Aeration, Freezing, Packaging, and Hardening

Aeration and freezing of the mixture occur in the scraped surface heat exchanger. During this stage, air is injected into the mixture to aerate it. This process leads to the relative incorporation of fat globules, formation of fat clusters, and encasement of air bubbles. As these fats crystallize, the air bubbles become more stable, and a relatively continuous network of fat is created. This network is crucial for the ice cream's texture, softness, resistance to melting, and maintaining its shape (avoiding wrinkling). It is important to note that maintaining a balance between fat, protein, and emulsifier is essential in ice cream production. This balance controls emulsion stability, facilitating a smoother aeration process and stability of air bubbles. If the protein content is too high, an overly stable emulsion is created, resulting in insufficient destabilization, leading to a moist ice cream with a coarse texture. Conversely, excessive emulsion instability (due to insufficient protein or excessive emulsifier) leads to excessive breakdown of fat globules, causing the fat clusters attached to each other to become large enough to be perceptible while eating, a phenomenon known as "buttering." The degree of fat instability becomes a significant factor in quality control. The outlet temperature of ice cream from continuous freezers varies between −6.11 and −5.56°C. Factors such as the overrun, tank pressure (approximately five atmospheres), output volume (around 3000 liters per hour), mixing speed (usually 200 revolutions per minute), and blade design are critical parameters in determining the outlet temperature. Freezing time depends on physical and mechanical factors, as well as mixture properties. Mechanical and physical factors include freezer type and design, cylinder wall conditions, blade speed, refrigerant temperature, refrigerant flow rate, amount of antifreezing oil on the external cylinder wall, volume expansion coefficient, and ice cream temperature during exit from the freezer (Figure 10.20). Additionally, certain mixture properties affecting freezing time include composition, freezing point, process method, and the type and quantity of flavor and aroma compounds. The mixture formula also significantly influences viscosity and the energy required to operate the freezer. Lowering the outlet temperature leads to smaller ice crystal sizes. The distribution of ice crystal sizes in regular ice cream is illustrated in Figure 10.21.

The injected air into the freezing tank passes through filters to ensure it is free from microbial contamination. Initially, the incoming air creates larger bubbles, but for producing high-quality ice cream, smaller bubbles need to be generated that will remain in the product. Agitation causes larger

Figure 10.20 Schematic of a continuous ice cream freezer.

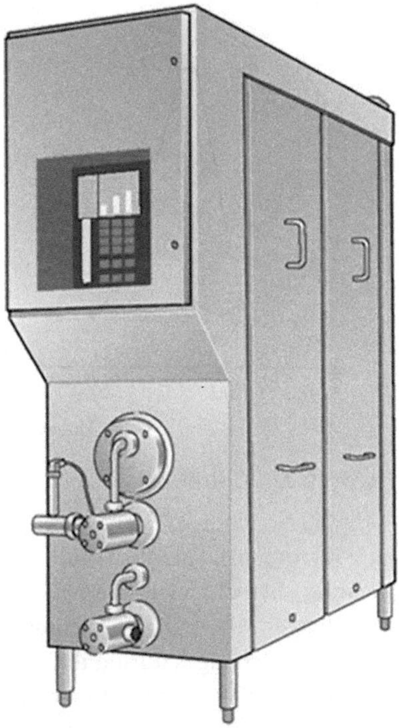

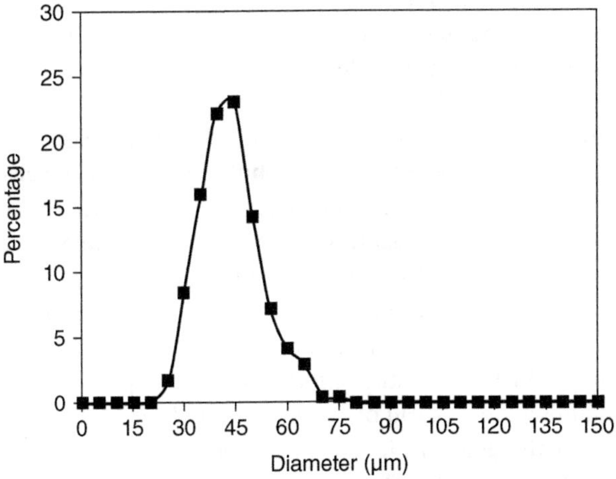

Figure 10.21 Distribution of ice crystal sizes in regular ice cream.

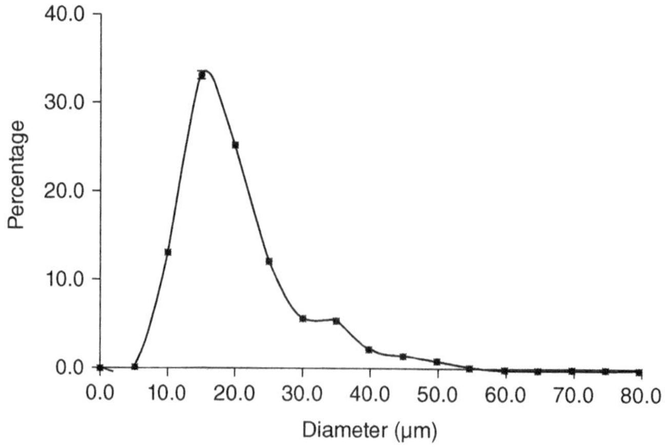

Figure 10.22 Distribution of air bubble sizes in regular ice cream.

bubbles to transform into a multitude of smaller bubbles. Although a strong shearing force can result in smaller air bubbles, if the dwell time in this stage is prolonged, the bubbles become even smaller. The way air bubble size distribution changes during the ice cream production process is illustrated in Figure 10.22 for regular ice cream.

There are two mechanisms for stabilizing air bubbles and preventing their coalescence in ice cream. The first involves the binding of proteins to the surface of air bubbles, reducing their surface tension. This occurs by positioning the hydrophilic end of the protein within the ice cream matrix and the hydrophobic end at the air bubble surface. As a result, the force caused by the phenomenon of disproportionation reduction diminishes, although it is not sufficient to eliminate it. The absorbed proteins, based on their arrangement, lead to the coalescence of fat globules. The second mechanism is related to the absorption of fat clusters. The relatively connected fat globules create three-dimensional structures that stabilize air bubbles and connect them to form a stable foam. This process does not occur if the fat is in liquid form because the fat globules coalesce into larger clusters resembling butter. Therefore, solid fat is necessary to create a proper foam structure. In modern ice cream production facilities, efforts are made to prevent secondary product contamination. Instead of air, nitrogen and carbon dioxide gases are used to achieve this goal. The ice cream freezer is a scraped surface cylinder, essentially a tubular heat exchanger, often oriented horizontally. It is surrounded by a refrigerant gas jacket (as shown in Figure 10.23). The refrigerant gas can be either ammonia or a refrigerant such as Freon. The mixture enters the freezer and, after approximately 30 seconds in

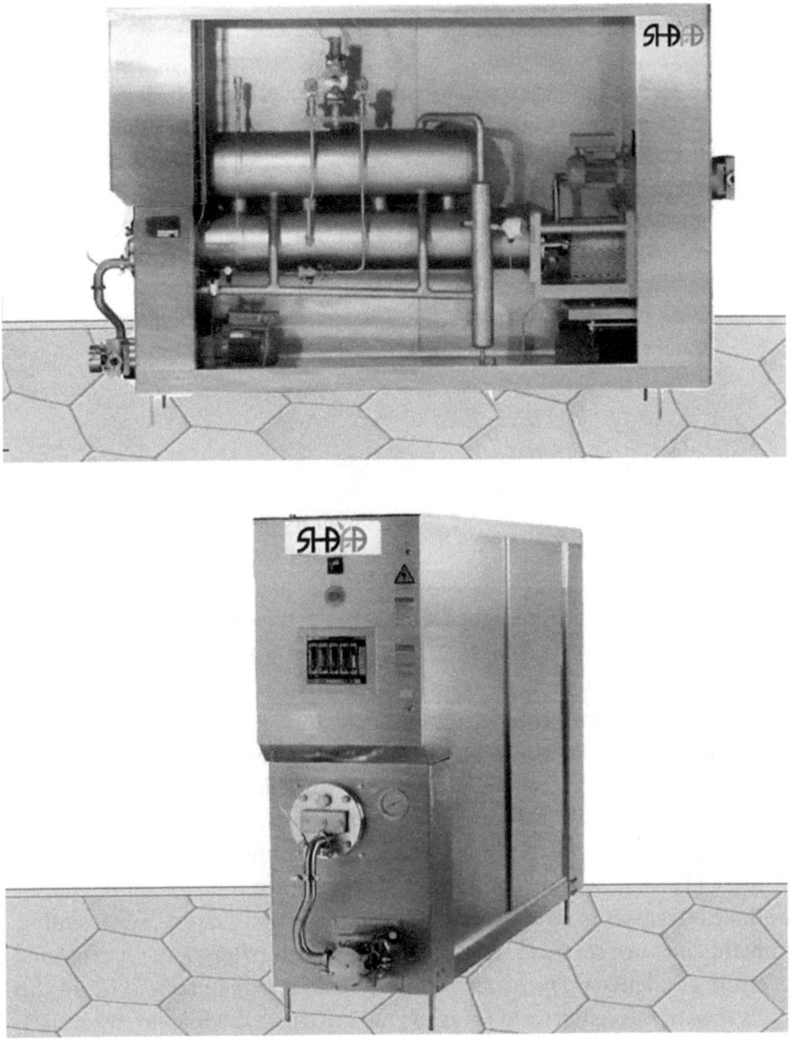

Figure 10.23 Internal diagram of a horizontal freezer for ice cream freezing.

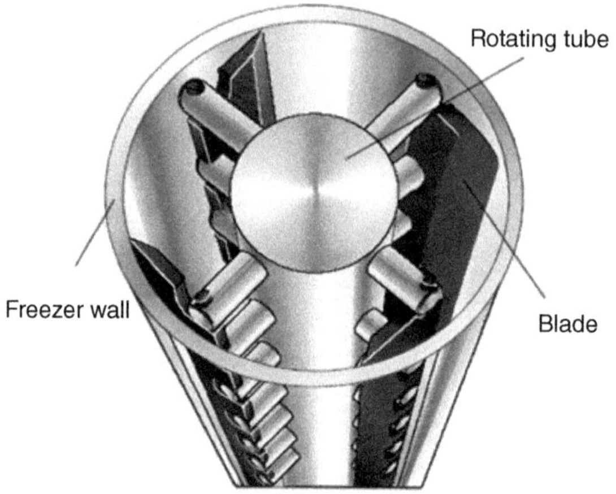

Figure 10.24 Internal diagram of a scraped surface heat exchanger system for ice cream freezing.

continuous freezers or 15–10 minutes in batch freezers, exits from the other end. During this process, about 50% of the mixture's water is frozen.

The freezer is equipped with scraping blades that shave off the frozen ice cream layer adhered to the inner wall of the cylinder and push it forward (see Figure 10.24). A rotating tube is positioned at the center of the cylinder, with the scraping blades located on its surface. This tube also features grooves through which air is injected into the mixture (see Figure 10.25). As the mixture comes into contact with the tank's wall, a thin layer of ice forms immediately and is promptly shaved off by the blades. Typically, there is about a 0.1-second interval between each shaving, so only an extremely thin layer of ice forms before each pass. Hence, maintaining the proper condition of these blades is crucial. Even if a thin layer of ice remains on the tank's wall, heat transfer is significantly reduced. The small ice crystals resulting from the shaving process are dispersed within the mixture. Two types of temperature gradients are formed within the tank: a radial gradient (from the walls toward the center) and an axial gradient (from the inlet to the outlet). Consequently, when the warmer ice crystals inside the mixture disperse, they melt and cool down the mixture. Near the entrance, all crystals melt, but as the mixture progresses one-third of its path in the tank, the temperature decreases enough for the remaining crystals to stay intact.

Ice cream contains a significant amount of air within its structure. Air constitutes approximately half of the volume of ice cream (see Figure 10.26). Aeration of ice cream leads to its lighter texture. Without aeration, ice cream would have a solid, cubical form. The amount of air present in ice cream is referred to as the overrun. Ice cream that emerges from the freezer is

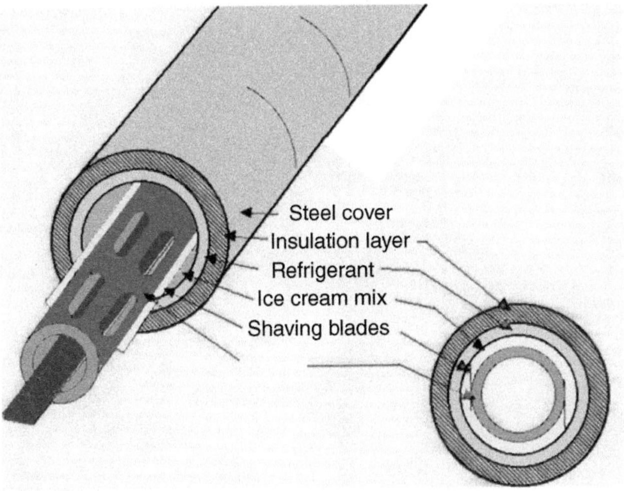

Figure 10.25 Components of a scraped surface heat exchanger system for ice cream freezing.

in a semifrozen and plastic (moldable) state. Immediately after exiting the freezer, specific additives like fruits, nuts, candies, and biscuits can be incorporated into it. In modern ice cream production systems, the ice cream is extruded, cut into desired shapes, and subsequently subjected to stick insertion (for stick-based ice cream) (see Figures 10.27–10.29, and 10.30).

The only difference between the fresh and soft ice creams consumed immediately after exiting the freezer, compared to hardened ice creams, is that soft ice cream is immediately packaged in a cone wrapper and made available for consumption. On the other hand, hardened ice creams are packaged in appropriate containers, and then solidified in a freezer or freezing tunnel. Sometimes, soft ice cream is also passed through a molding machine after exiting the freezer to be frozen in various shapes. In Figure 10.29, a general overview of the stick ice cream production process is presented. This process involves stages such as filling, partial freezing, stick insertion, complete freezing, product extraction, washing, rinsing, and sanitization. The hardening process involves placing ice cream packages in a freezing tunnel with a flow of extremely cold air at temperatures around −30 to −40°C. As a result, another portion of the unfrozen water present in the texture freezes (Figures 10.31 and 10.32). During the process of hardening, the crystals can grow through two methods. One is by freezing more water, producing larger ice crystals, a process known as ice crystal propagation. The other method is recrystallization, where smaller crystals combine to form larger ones without changing the overall amount of ice. The lower

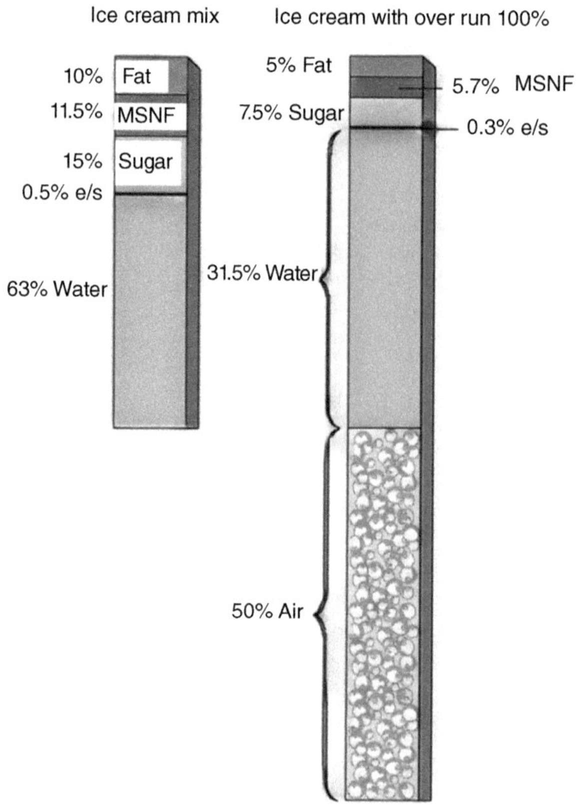

Figure 10.26 Comparison of ice cream mix components with the final product.

the temperature, the slower the crystallization process occurs. Therefore, to minimize recrystallization and promote ice crystal propagation, the hardening process should be conducted as rapidly as possible. In recrystallization, two phenomena, Ostwald ripening and accretion, play a significant role. Ostwald ripening is more influential at the beginning of the hardening process when the volume of the ice phase is low. On the other hand, agglomeration becomes crucial when the amount of ice increases due to ice crystal multiplication. During agglomeration, the distance between two crystals decreases, and they come into contact with each other during growth. It is important to note that during the hardening process, no new crystals are formed because the energy required for nucleation is lost due to the cooling process.

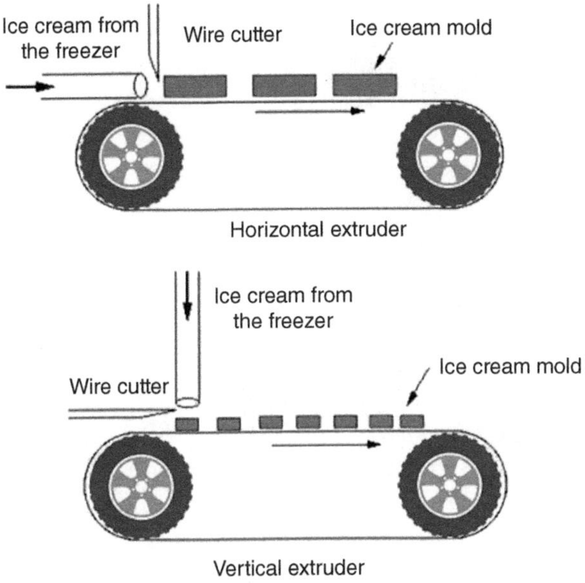

Figure 10.27 Diagram of horizontal and vertical extruder machines.

Figure 10.28 Vertical extruder machine.

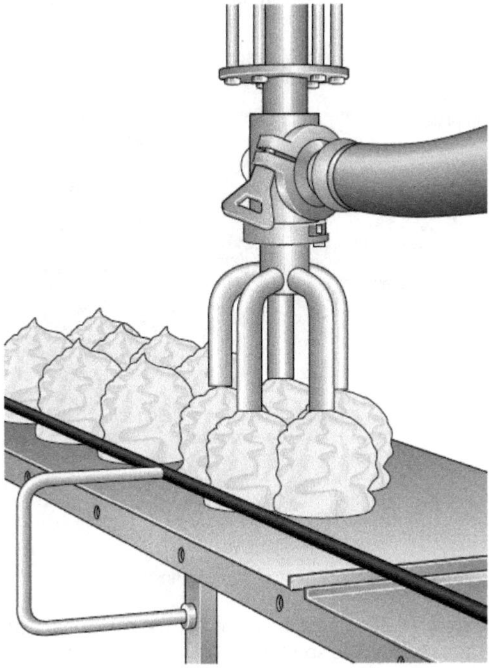

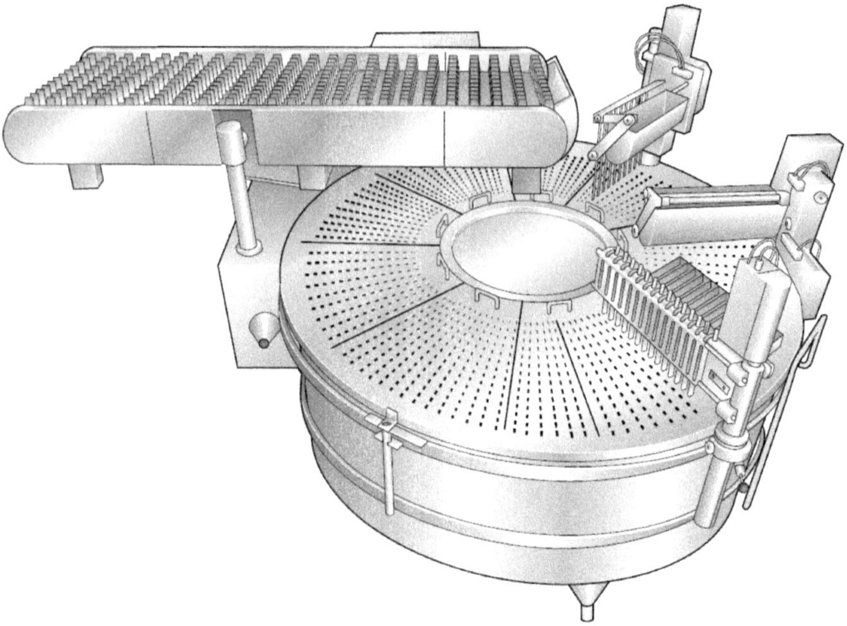

Figure 10.29 Ice cream bar freezer (Tetra Pak Processing Systems).

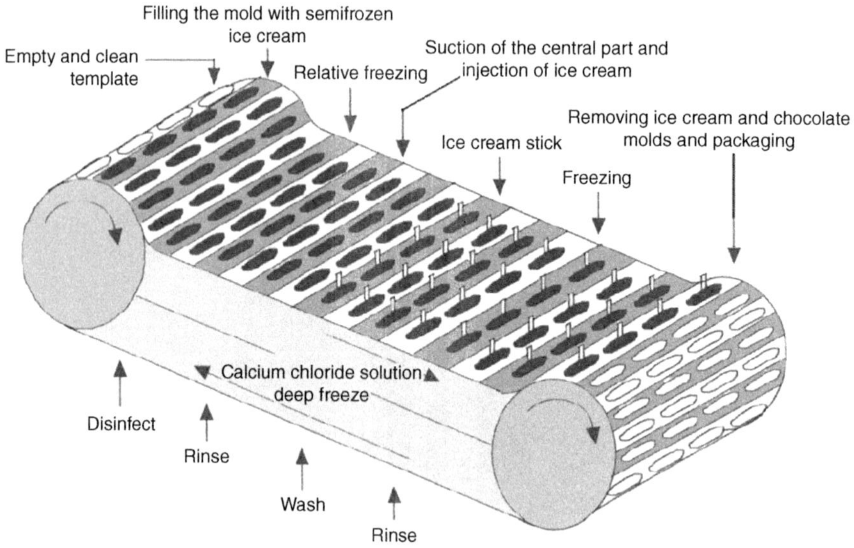

Figure 10.30 Mechanism of the ice cream bar freezer (Molds are placed in the calcium chloride solution).

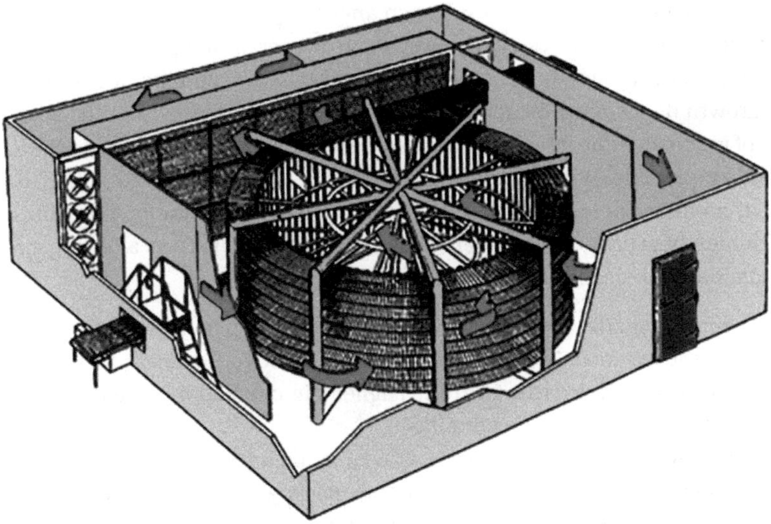

Figure 10.31 Spiral hardening tunnel for ice cream production.

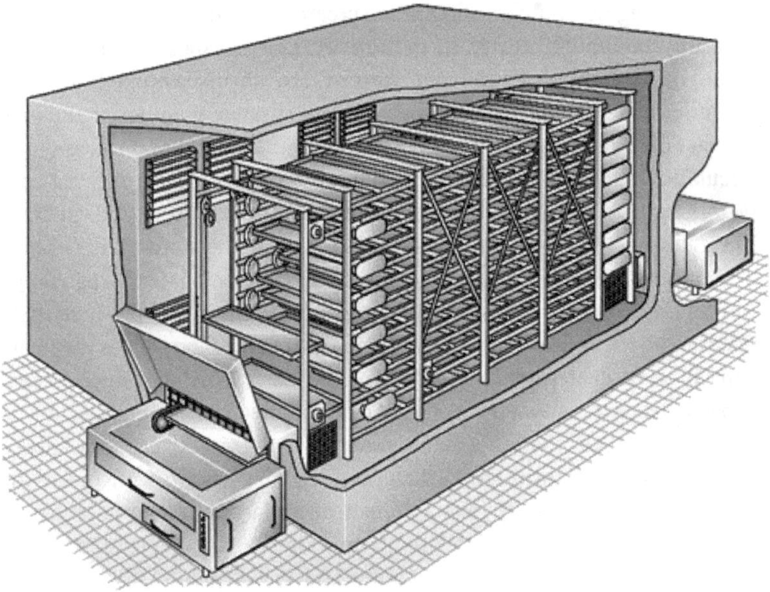

Figure 10.32 Hardening tunnel for ice cream production (Tetra Pak Processing Systems).

At temperatures below −25°C, ice cream can be stored indefinitely without the occurrence of ice crystal growth. However, at temperatures above this range, the growth of ice crystals becomes possible, and the rate of crystal growth depends on the temperature of the freezer. This affects the shelf life of ice cream. The freezing speed of ice cream in the tunnel should be relatively rapid. Therefore, in freezing tunnels, very cold air (around −40°C) is used, circulated at high speed (forced circulation by fans), and freezer plates with high heat conductivity coefficients are employed. Factors affecting ice cream hardening include:

1. **Tunnel-freezing temperature:** The lower the tunnel temperature, the faster the ice cream will harden, resulting in a softer texture.
2. **Airflow speed in the tunnel:** Higher air circulation speeds in the tunnel increase heat transfer rates.
3. **Initial ice cream temperature:** Colder ice cream placed in the freezing tunnel hardens more quickly. Therefore, packaging operations should be carried out rapidly, and the time between transferring ice cream from the freezer to the tunnel should be minimized.
4. **Container size:** Smaller ice cream containers harden more quickly. Thus, packaging and cartoning of ice cream containers should be done after the hardening process in the tunnel. This is especially important when ice cream packages and cartons are shrink-wrapped. Larger amounts of ice cream are compacted into smaller volumes, reducing the rate of hardening. In summary, freezing speed, temperature, and air circulation play crucial roles in the hardening of ice cream, and various factors need to be optimized to achieve the desired texture and quality. The required duration for ice cream to stay in the hardening tunnel depends on several factors, including the coefficient of expansion, formulation, exit temperature, and the final amount of product that needs to be packaged. A higher coefficient of expansion reduces the heat capacity and heat transfer capacity of the ice cream. A reduced heat capacity leads to a smaller amount of heat that needs to be removed from the ice cream. On the other hand, reduced heat transfer capacity slows down the heat removal rate. Thus, these two factors work inversely to each other. Heat capacity has a greater effect, and a higher coefficient of expansion leads to a shorter hardening time. The composition of ice cream can also affect its freezing point and, consequently, the speed of hardening. The arrangement of ice cream items in the tunnel affects air circulation and the rate of hardening. Items must be positioned

to allow easy air circulation without creating pockets of stagnant air. Maintenance and care of the operator are also crucial. The operator should be free from frost as frost acts as a thermal insulator. The type of packaging material also affects hardening speed. Although materials like Styrofoam or corrugated cardboard can prevent heat shock after hardening, they reduce heat transfer rates if used before hardening, resulting in a longer hardening time. Therefore, using such packaging (cartons) for products right out of the freezer is not practical. After hardening, ice cream is stored in a cold room with temperatures ranging from −25 to −35°C before being sent to the market. In distribution, the key task is to maintain the cold chain to ensure the product reaches the consumer with appropriate quality. It is evident that most of the quality degradation of ice cream occurs during the distribution phase, and in developing countries, maintaining the cold chain is crucial, indicating the advancement of a country. A schematic of an ice cream production line with capacities of 500–5000 liters per hour is shown in Figures 10.33 and 10.34, respectively (Homayouni et al. 2008; Homayouni 2008; Homayouni 2009).

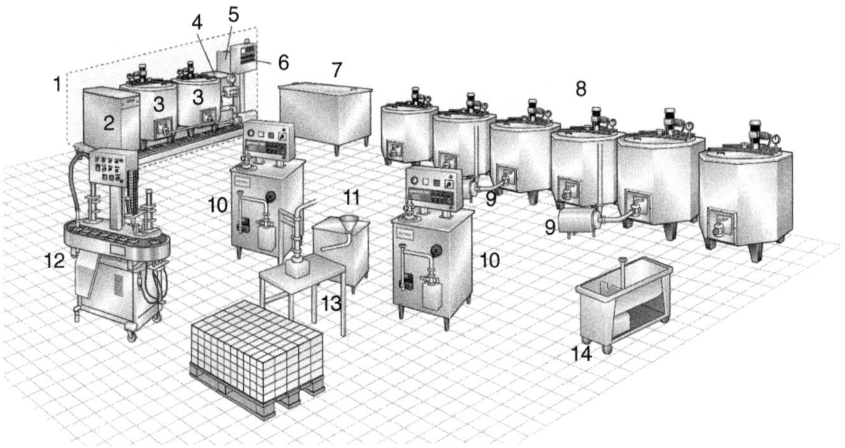

Figure 10.33 Schematic of an ice cream production line with a capacity of 500 liters per hour 1: Ice cream mix preparation module, 2: Water heater, 3: Mixing and processing tank, 4: Homogenizer, 5: Plate heat exchanger, 6: Control panel, 7: Cooling water unit, 8: Ageing tanks, 9: Discharge pumps, 10: Continuous freezers, 11: Ripple pump, 12: Roto-filler, 13: Can filler, 14: Manual CIP unit (Tetra Pak Processing Systems).

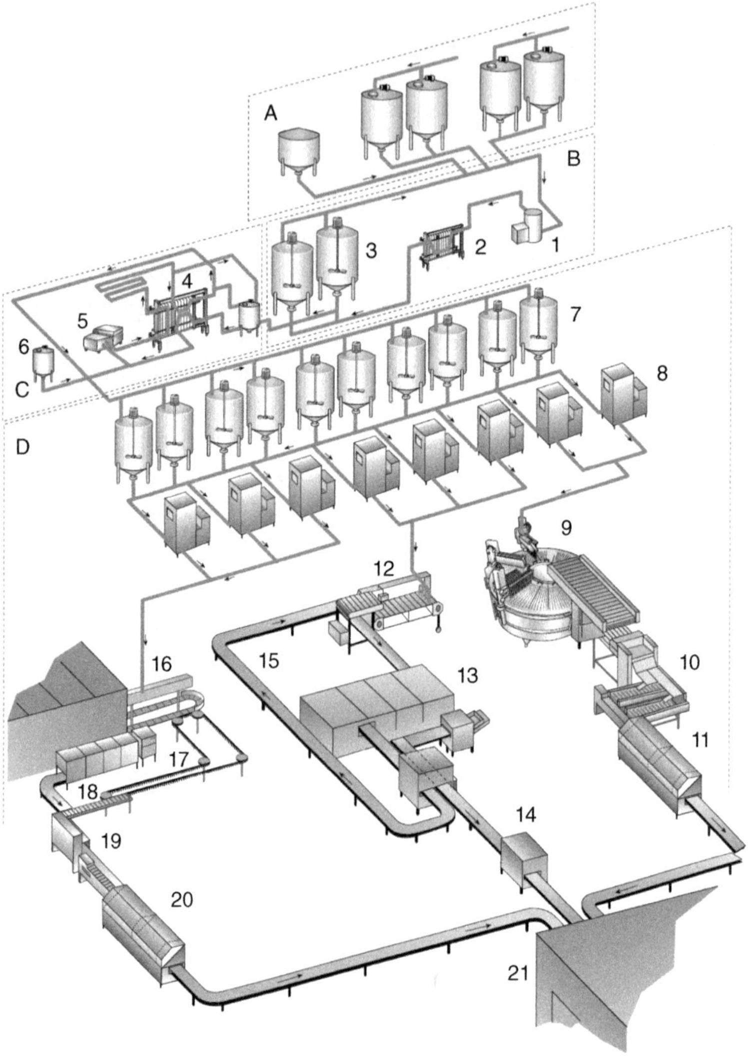

Figure 10.34 Schematic of an ice cream production line with a capacity of 5000 liters per hour A: Raw material storage, B: Dissolving of ingredients and mixing, C: Pasteurization, homogenization, and fat standardization of the mix, D: Ice cream production plant, 1: Mixing unit, 2: Plate heat exchanger, 3: Mixing tanks (at least two for continuous processing), 4: Plate heat exchanger, 5: Homogenizer, 6: Tank for AMF or vegetable fat, 7: Ageing tanks, 8: Continuous freezers, 9: Bar freezer, 10: Wrapping and stacking unit, 11: Cartoning unit, 12: Cup/cone filler, 13: Hardening tunnel, 14: Cartoning line, 15: Return conveyor for empty trays, 16: Tray tunnel extruder, 17: Chocolate enrobing unit, 18: Cooling tunnel, 19: Wrapping unit, 20: Cartoning unit, 21: Cold storage (Tetra Pak Processing Systems).

References

Homayouni, A. (2008). Effect of microencapsulation and resistant starch on the probiotic survival and sensory properties of synbiotic ice cream. PhD thesis, University of Tehran, Iran.

Homayouni, A., Azizi, A., Ehsani, M.R., and Yarmand, M.S. (2008). Effect of microencapsulation and resistant starch on the probiotic survival and sensory properties of synbiotic ice cream. *Food Chemistry* 111 (1): 50–55.

Homayouni, A. (2009). *Therapeutical Effects of Functional Probiotic, Prebiotic and Synbiotic Foods*. Tabriz, Iran: Tabriz University of Medical Sciences.

Tetra Pak Processing Systems AB (1995). *S-221 86 Lund, Dairy Processing Handbook*. Sweden.

11

Ice Cream as a Probiotic/Prebiotic Delivery Vehicle

11.1 Ice Cream as a Probiotic/Prebiotic Delivery Vehicle

Probiotic ice cream can be created by introducing probiotic bacteria into both fermented and unfermented ice cream mixes. Ice cream serves as an excellent vehicle for delivering these beneficial microorganisms into the human diet, as supported by several studies. Lactic acid bacteria, specifically *Lactobacillus* and *Bifidobacterium*, are commonly used as probiotics in fermented dairy products. Probiotic ice cream, among various frozen dairy products containing live probiotics, is gaining popularity due to its neutral pH. The near-neutral pH of nonfermented ice cream, which is close to seven, creates a favorable environment for probiotic bacteria to thrive (Homayouni et al. 2008). The high total solids content in ice cream, encompassing both fat and milk solids, provides a protective shield for probiotic bacteria. However, the efficiency of added probiotics depends on factors such as dosage, the type of dairy product, the presence of air, and low temperatures (Homayouni, 2009). To meet their therapeutic potential, these probiotic bacteria must remain viable throughout the product's shelf-life and withstand the conditions of the gastrointestinal tract. The IDF recommends that a minimum of 10^7 probiotic bacterial cells should be alive per gram of product at the time of consumption. Studies indicate that probiotic bacteria may not survive in sufficient numbers in frozen dairy products unless appropriate measures are taken to mitigate freeze injury and oxygen toxicity. Figure 11.1 illustrates the factors influencing probiotic survival in ice cream. The methods employed to enhance probiotic survival depend on the type of food product. One crucial method involves selecting probiotic strains that are inherently resistant to the conditions encountered during production, storage, and passage through the gastrointestinal tract (Homayouni et.al. 2012).

Probiotic Ice Cream: Science and Technology, First Edition. Aziz Homayouni-Rad.

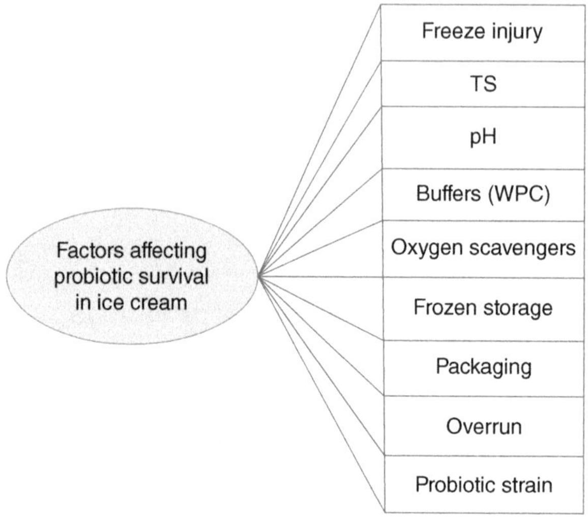

Figure 11.1 Factors affecting probiotic survival in ice cream.

Another effective approach is to modify the production and storage conditions to enhance probiotic survival rates. Adjusting the physical environment in which probiotics are produced and stored can make a significant difference. A relatively new and promising method for increasing probiotic survival is through microencapsulation. This technique involves enveloping bacterial cells with a protective coating, isolating them from the harsh conditions of the product and the gastrointestinal tract. This protective encapsulation has the potential to reduce cell loss and, consequently, extend the shelf-life of probiotic cultures in frozen dairy products (Homayouni, 2008). The selection of suitable probiotic strains plays a crucial role in their ability to survive the simulated conditions encountered in ice cream, such as high sucrose concentrations, elevated oxygen levels, freezing and storage temperatures, as well as both acidic (simulating the gastric environment) and alkaline conditions (simulating the intestinal environment). Microencapsulation of probiotics offers an additional layer of protection against these challenging conditions, further enhancing their viability and potential health benefits. Nonfermented probiotic ice cream stands out among dairy products with live probiotics as an effective vehicle for delivering live probiotic cells to the human intestinal tract. This suitability arises from its neutral pH and elevated total solids content, both of which offer a protective environment for probiotic bacteria. However, it is important to note that the harsh conditions associated with ice cream formulation and manufacturing, such as high osmotic pressure, varying oxygen levels due to overrun, and the properties of packaging materials, as well as the freezing and storage temperatures, can potentially pose challenges to probiotic survival. Additionally, the acidic and alkaline conditions within the human intestinal tract may also influence probiotic viability. This study provides a comprehensive review of the factors that impact probiotic survival in ice cream, shedding light on the complexities of maintaining probiotic effectiveness in this particular dairy product (Homayouni et al. 2012). Two variations of synbiotic ice cream, both containing 1% resistant starch and featuring *Lactobacillus casei (Lc-01)* and *Bifidobacterium lactis (Bb-12)*, were produced. The viability of *L. casei* and *B. lactis* was observed over a 180-day storage period at −20°C. In the initial ice cream mixture, the viable cell count of *L. casei* and *B. lactis* in their free state was 5.1 × 10^9 and 4.1 × 10^9 CFU/mL on the first day. After 180 days of storage at −20°C, these counts decreased to 4.2 × 10^6 and 1.1 × 10^7 CFU/mL, respectively. However, when the mentioned probiotic bacteria were encapsulated in calcium alginate beads, their survival rate increased by approximately 30% during the same storage period at the same temperature. In summary, the findings suggest that encapsulation significantly enhances the survival rate of probiotic bacteria in ice cream, extending its shelf life. The incorporation of encapsulated probiotics did not have any notable impact on the sensory characteristics of nonfermented ice cream, where resistant starch served as the prebiotic component. This research underscores the significant enhancement in the survival of probiotic bacteria achievable through encapsulation when incorporated into ice cream. Dairy products like ice cream and frozen desserts can effectively serve as carriers for delivering probiotic bacteria to the human gut. The substantial total solids content in ice cream, including fat and milk solids, offers a protective environment for these probiotic bacteria. During the first month, the loss in viable *L. casei* and *B. lactis* cells in their free state amounted to only 0.7 and 0.4 log, respectively, whereas in the encapsulated state, it was 0.3 and 0.2 log. Over the subsequent five months, the decline continued, resulting in a total reduction of 2.7 and 2.5 log in the free state and 1.1 and 0.5 log in the encapsulated state, respectively. After six months, there was a final decrease of 3.4 and 2.9 logs in the free state of *L. casei* and *B. lactis*, compared to 1.4 and 0.7 log in the encapsulated state. At the conclusion of a three-month storage period, which corresponds to the typical shelf life of ice cream, all types of ice cream contained between 10^8 and 10^9 colony-forming units (CFUs) per gram, exceeding the IDF's recommended count of 10^7 cfu/g. This suggests that the high initial probiotic count can maintain the recommended level in the final product. Additional research is necessary to assess the protective impact of microencapsulation on probiotic survival within the gastrointestinal tract (Homayouni et al. 2008). The surging demand for functional foods has prompted scientists to investigate the production and preservation conditions of these products. In this context, fermented soy ice cream containing *L. casei* ssp. casei CRL-431 was crafted using soy milk powder, and an assessment of the product's physicochemical, rheological, and sensory attributes was carried out. Over a 180-day storage period at −24°C, the survival of *L. casei* was continuously monitored. Comparing the fermented soy ice cream to the control sample (soy ice cream), several noteworthy differences were observed. There was a significant increase ($P < 0.05$) in acidity, reaching 0.455 ± 0.005 °D, as well as overrun, which reached $42.57 \pm 8.5\%$, and relative density, measured at 1.1319 ± 0.0002 cP, in the fermented soy ice cream. However, the viscosity of the control sample was higher than that of the fermented soy ice cream after 30 minutes, with values of 1121 cP and 1104.32 cP, respectively. Notably, there was no significant reduction in the enumeration of probiotics in the fermented soy ice cream throughout the study. The viable cell count of *L. casei* started at 3.1×106 cfu/g before freezing, ultimately decreasing to 1×106 cfu/g by the study's end. Additionally, the sensory attributes of the fermented soy ice cream exhibited significant improvements due to the fermentation process. One of the most notable discoveries from this research is that fermented soy ice cream has the potential to enhance the viability and stability of *L. casei* for a duration of up to 180 days. Additionally, the study's outcomes indicate that fermentation can lead to improvements in the physicochemical and sensory characteristics of soy ice cream. Collectively, these findings imply that fermented soy ice cream, on the whole, can serve as an effective medium for delivering *L. casei* to the human gastrointestinal tract. It is advisable to further investigate the impact of production and preservation conditions on other functional components present in fermented soy ice cream, such as isoflavones. Additionally, it is suggested to explore the viability of different strains of probiotics under the preservation conditions specific to fermented soy ice cream (Homayouni et al. 2020).

11.2 Challenges Toward Adding Probiotics into Ice Cream

A significant challenge in the production of probiotic products, particularly functional foods, lies in identifying a suitable carrier for these microorganisms. This research has effectively demonstrated that soy ice cream, characterized by its neutral pH, elevated total solids content, and the presence of soy-based growth factors, can serve as an ideal medium for delivering *L. casei*. Furthermore, the substantial number of viable probiotic cells remaining in this dessert even after prolonged storage at freezing temperatures highlights the robustness of *L. casei*, which can withstand low temperatures, cold shock, high sucrose levels, and oxygen content (Homayouni et al. 2012). This study has unveiled key properties of probiotic soy ice cream and its potential applications in the food industry. Consequently, probiotic soy ice cream emerges as a promising ingredient with significant nutritional value. Probiotics are defined as live microorganisms which, when administered in adequate amounts, confer a health benefit on the host. Prebiotics are nondigestible substances that provide a beneficial physiological effect on the host by selectively stimulating the favorable growth or activity of a limited number of indigenous bacteria. A food product containing both probiotics and prebiotics is called synbiotic or functional food. There is a synergic effect between probiotics and prebiotics in synbiotic products. Prebiotic compounds are consumed by probiotics as a carbon or energy source in the colon. This results in an increase of probiotic count and a reduction of pathogen microorganisms in the gut. Probiotic bacteria have been incorporated into fermented and nonfermented ice cream which is an ideal vehicle for delivery of these organisms in the human diet. *Lactobacillus* and *Bifidobacterium* are the most common species of lactic acid bacteria used as probiotics for the production of fermented dairy products. Among the frozen dairy products with live probiotics, synbiotic ice cream is also gaining popularity for its neutral pH. The pH of nonfermented ice cream is closer to 7 and this provides possibility for satisfactory survival of probiotic bacteria. The high total solids level in ice cream including the fat and milk solids provides protection for the probiotic bacteria. Because the efficiency of added probiotic bacteria depends on dose level, type of dairy foods, presence of air and low temperature, their viability must be maintained throughout the product's shelf-life and they must survive the gut environment. The therapeutic value of live probiotic bacteria is more than unviable cells; therefore, IDF suggests that a minimum of 10^7 probiotic bacterial cells should be alive at the time of consumption per gram of product. Studies indicate, however, that the bacteria may not survive in high enough numbers when incorporated into frozen dairy products unless a suitable method is used against freeze injury and oxygen toxicity. The methods of increasing probiotic survival depend on the type of food products. Selection of resistant probiotic strains to tolerate production, storage and gastrointestinal tract conditions, is one of the important methods. Another way is to adjust the conditions of production and storage for higher survival rates. The physical protection of probiotics by microencapsulation is a new method for increasing the survival of probiotics. Encapsulation helps to isolate the bacterial cells from the adverse environment of the product and gastrointestinal tract, thus potentially reducing cell loss.

Encapsulation thus may enhance the shelf-life of probiotic cultures in frozen dairy products.

To enhance the viability and survival of probiotic bacteria in non-fermented ice cream, first we must select appropriate probiotic strains which are able to survive simulated conditions of ice cream (high sucrose concentrations, high oxygen, refrigeration, and freezing temperatures), acidic (to simulate gastric), and alkaline conditions (to simulate intestinal). Secondly, we should microencapsulate the probiotics to further protect these bacteria from the mentioned conditions. In the first step, the growth and survival rate of *Lactobacillus acidophilus, L. casei, B. lactis,* and *Bifidobacterium longum* in varying amounts of sucrose concentrations (10, 15, 20, and 25%), oxygen scavenging components (0.05% L-cysteine and 0.05% L-ascorbate) and low temperatures (4°C and −20°C) during different periods of time (1, 2, and 3 months) in MRS-broth medium was evaluated. All of the stress factors investigated have been able to affect the growth and survival of related probiotics. The results have proved that it is possible to select the appropriate probiotic strains for use in ice cream. In conclusion, a comparison with other probiotic strains revealed that *L. casei (Lc01)* and *B. lactis (Bb12)* had the highest resistance to simulated acidic, alkaline, and ice cream conditions, making them suitable probiotic strains for use in ice cream. In the second step, a modified microencapsulation method based on emulsion technique was investigated. The objectives of the present study were first to develop a method for producing alginate microspheres containing viable probiotic bacteria with diameters below 100 μm, and second, to optimize the microencapsulation process yield by using the varying amounts of lecithin (0, 0.2, 0.4, and 1%) and calcium chloride solution (100 and 200 mL). In addition, the effect of surfactant type on the microencapsulation process yield was investigated. Recent study has indicated that it is possible to control the alginate microsphere size by using high stirring speed (400 rpm for 20 minutes) of emulsion and produce spherical beads in the range of 10–30 micrometers. This gives a smooth texture when the beads are incorporated into products. It was shown that the microencapsulation process yield of alginate beads may be dependent on the surfactant type and concentration as well as the volume of calcium chloride solution. Tween 80 had better ability than lecithin in alginate bead production and a higher volume of $CaCl_2$ solution resulted in high microencapsulation process yield. In the third step, survival of free and microencapsulated *L. casei (Lc01)* and *B. lactis (Bb12)* in synbiotic ice cream containing resistant starch as a prebiotic substance was investigated. This study was undertaken to evaluate the feasibility of incorporating resistant starch into bead coating and ice cream formulation. The survival of microencapsulated and free cultures in ice cream was studied over a period of 180 days during storage at −20°C. This study indicated that encapsulation can significantly improve the survival of probiotic bacteria in ice cream. There was a loss of only 0.7 and 0.4 log in the free state of *L. casei* and *B. lactis*, respectively, and 0.3 and 0.2 log in the encapsulated state over the first month and 2.7 and 2.5 log in the free state and 1.1 and 0.5 log in the encapsulated state over the subsequent 5 months, respectively. The final count after six months showed a 3.4 and 2.9 log decrease in the free state of *L. casei* and *B. lactis*, respectively, compared to 1.4 and 0.7 log in the encapsulated state, respectively. After one month, microencapsulated probiotics in alginate beads survived 30% more than encapsulated bacteria. The numbers of viable probiotic bacteria in all types of ice cream were between 10^8 and 10^9 CFU/g by the three months, higher than that recommended by the IDF (10^7 CFU/g). These results showed that the high initial number of encapsulated probiotics can provide the required standard in the final product (Homayouni 2008).

References

Homayouni, A. (2008). Effect of microencapsulation and resistant starch on the probiotic survival and sensory properties of synbiotic ice cream. PhD thesis, University of Tehran, Iran.

Homayouni, A. (2009). *Therapeutical Effects of Functional Probiotic, Prebiotic and Synbiotic Foods*. Tabriz, Iran: Tabriz University of Medical Sciences.

Homayouni, A., Azizi, A., Ehsani, M.R., and Yarmand, M.S. (2008). Effect of microencapsulation and resistant starch on the probiotic survival and sensory properties of synbiotic ice cream. *Food Chemistry* 111 (1): 50–55.

Homayouni, A., Azizi, A., Javadi, M. et al. (2012). Factors influencing probiotic survival in ice cream a review. *International Journal of Dairy Science* 7 (1): 1–10.

Homayouni, A., Rezaei, M.R., Norouzi, S. et al. (2020). Soy ice cream as a carrier for efficient delivering of *Lactobacillus casei*. *Nutrition & Food Science* 51 (1): 61–70.

Part III

Quality Control

12

Physicochemical, Rheological, and Microbial Properties of Probiotic Ice Cream

12.1 The Properties of Probiotic Ice Cream

Ice cream is a complex food colloid, comprising an unfrozen serum phase, ice crystals, fat globules, and air bubbles. Its primary components include fat, nonfat milk solids, sucrose, stabilizers, and emulsifiers. The creation of this structure involves several manufacturing steps, including mixing, pasteurization, homogenization, aging, freezing, and hardening. Broadly speaking, analytical techniques for ice cream analysis fall into three categories: chemical (covering both volatile and nonvolatile compounds), physical (encompassing rheological and color analysis), and structural analysis. This study aims to provide an overview of the novel methods employed in ice cream analysis (Homayouni et al. 2018). In some cases, probiotic bacteria may also be added to the ice cream (Homayouni et al. 2008; Homayouni et al. 2012). The size of ice crystals and air bubbles typically falls within the range of 20–50 μm. Air bubbles are partially coated with fat globules, and these fat globules, in turn, are enveloped by a protein/emulsifier layer. The serum phase consists of sucrose, lactose, glucose, high molecular weight polysaccharides, and probiotic cells within a freeze-concentrated solution (Homayouni et al. 2008). During the homogenization process of fat, proteins and emulsifiers occupy interfacial spaces, creating an emulsion in the mixture. Following the crystallization and homogenization of fat, the fat globule membrane reorganizes itself into a state of minimal free dynamism. This resulting emulsion then undergoes whipping and ice crystal formation during the dynamic freezing process. These processes contribute to the development of the four main structural components of the frozen product: a network of partially coalesced fat surrounding the air bubbles, a discontinuous foam, ice crystals, and a continuous, unfrozen aqueous solution. This chapter aims to provide a review of the innovative methods used for analyzing the structure

Probiotic Ice Cream: Science and Technology, First Edition. Aziz Homayouni-Rad.

of ice cream. In general, these analysis methods can be categorized into three groups: chemical (covering volatile and nonvolatile compounds), physical (including rheological and color analysis), and structural analysis. Ice cream analysis can employ a range of advanced methods, tailored to the specific components being studied, such as ice crystals, fat globules, air bubbles, probiotic cells, sucrose, vanillin, and hydrocolloids. This chapter highlights that chemical, physical, and structural analysis methods are all suitable for examining ice cream.

12.2 Physical Properties

Ice cream mixture consists of two phases: water and fat. Carbohydrates and serum proteins in the aqueous phase are either in solution or in colloidal suspension. The fat phase exists in an emulsified state. The important characteristics of ice cream mixture include surface tension and interfacial tension, stability, density, acidity, surface adsorption, freezing point, and whippability, which will be discussed in detail below.

12.2.1 Surface Tension and Interfacial Tension

"Surface tension" refers to the force generated by the attraction between molecules at the surface of a liquid. As the intermolecular attraction increases, the surface tension increases, and as the attraction between liquid molecules decreases, surface tension decreases. "Interfacial tension" is the force involved at the interface between two liquids or between a liquid and a gas. Interfacial tension changes based on the type, orientation, and number of molecules present. Surface tension and interfacial tension are interrelated since conditions that cause stress on a liquid surface can induce stress at the boundary between two liquids as well. The values of surface tension and interfacial tension vary inversely with each other. Surface tension is defined as the work required to increase the surface area by one unit. The unit of surface tension (γ) is energy per unit area and is expressed as N/m or J/m^2. The surface tension of pure water at 20°C is approximately 72.8 mN/m. Water has a much higher surface tension compared to most other liquids. Surface tension is defined as the interface between a liquid and air, while the term "interfacial tension" is used for the boundary between two phases, such as oil and water. Surface tension is measured using a tensiometer device. This device records the maximum force needed to pull a loop or a platinum plate out of a confined liquid. For measuring the surface tension of an ice cream mixture, the Du Nouy method is commonly used (Figure 12.1). In this method, the maximum force required to detach

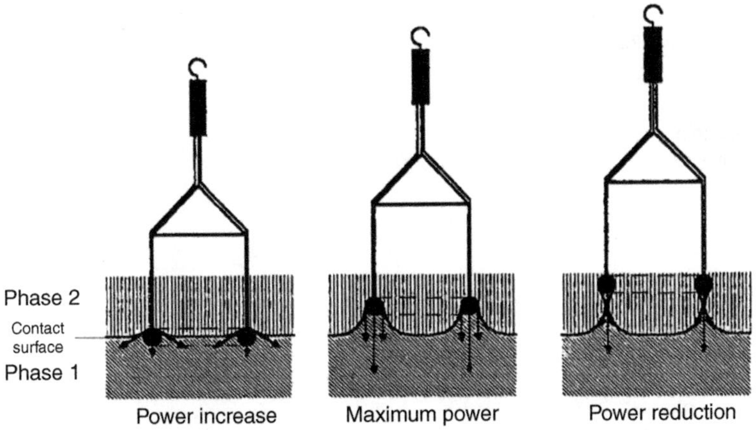

Figure 12.1 Steps of surface tension measurement in ice cream mixture.

a ring or a platinum plate from the ice cream mixture at the common interface of the mixture and air is recorded. Surface-active compounds like emulsifiers decrease the surface tension. This can result in weakening the body and causing coarseness in the final product. Studies have shown that the interfacial tension of oil-in-water emulsions containing mono- and diglycerides and polysorbates is closely related to the degree of protein extraction from the interfacial layer. The presence of these compounds in the ice cream mixture before homogenization significantly reduces the interfacial tension between the phases (Figure 12.2). The surface adsorption of emulsifiers to the air–water interface can be evaluated by measuring surface tension. This is because emulsifiers have a much greater effect on surface tension than proteins. Additionally, this method allows for the investigation of the mechanism of emulsifier attachment.

12.2.2 Stability

The stability of the ice cream mixture depends on the resistance of milk proteins in the colloidal suspension and fat emulsions against separation. The destabilization of the mixture can lead to the following outcomes:

(a) Aggregation and sedimentation of protein particles.
(b) Separation of whey from the mixture.
(c) Syrup separation during freezing.

Factors such as acidity, salt concentration, fat-to-nonfat solid ratio, bound water content, heat treatment, homogenization, aging time, and freezing affect the stability of the mixture. In a homogenized mixture, fat globules

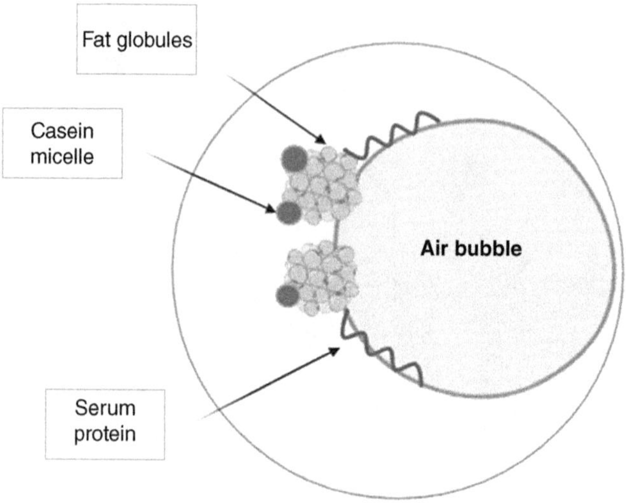

Figure 12.2 Arrangement of proteins in fat globule membranes and air bubbles.

are surrounded by a layer of milk proteins. This layer has a thickness of around 0.3 microns, which is larger than the size of fat globules. This layer can interact with water, leading to increased particle cohesion and, consequently, improved stability. During freezing, fat globules can aggregate and cluster due to churning and the thickening property of freezing. This process reduces fat stability.

12.2.3 Density

Density, also known as specific gravity, is the mass per unit volume of the ice cream mixture and can be measured using a densitometer or the pycnometer method. The density of ice cream mixture typically varies within the range of 1.09–1.1 kilograms per liter (kg/L).

12.2.4 Acidity

The acidity of an ice cream mixture is related to the amount of nonfat solids present in the mixture before titration. By multiplying the nonfat solids content by a factor of 0.017, the acidity of the mixture can be determined. Therefore, a mixture containing 11% nonfat solids will have a titratable acidity of 0.178%. It is evident that acidity increases with higher nonfat solids content. The pH of the mixture is also influenced by its composition. Colloidal suspensions are sensitive to changes in pH and salt concentration. The acidity of ice cream is around 6.3. High acidity is undesirable as it leads to increased viscosity, reduced overrun (aeration), undesirable taste, and mixture instability. Additionally, it accelerates changes in protein nature during mixing and pasteurization, contributing to the coarsening and icy texture of the ice cream. Low acidity also has an undesirable impact on the taste of ice cream.

12.2.5 Surface Adsorption

Surface adsorption refers to the absorption of molecules onto surfaces formed within the ice cream mixture. These absorbed molecules create a new layer on the surfaces. This process reduces the interfacial tension between the components of the mixture. The materials that are adsorbed onto a surface are arranged according to their ability to reduce the interfacial tension on that specific surface. For example, proteins by being adsorbed onto the surface of fat globules can reduce interfacial tension (Figure 12.2). This effect is particularly pronounced in mixtures treated with the enzyme protease chymosin, as proteins undergo hydrolysis in this case, resulting in lower molecular weight and lighter components that are easily absorbed onto the surfaces of fat globules. Emulsifying agents with a low HLB value can also be adsorbed onto the surface of fat globules, thereby reducing interfacial tension. From the information mentioned earlier, it can be inferred that molecules with higher molecular activity and smaller sizes act as strong reducers of interfacial tension. In other words, molecules with greater ability to be adsorbed onto a surface can displace previously adsorbed molecules and take their place in the surface layer.

12.2.6 Freezing Point

The freezing point is one of the characteristics of a mixture that depends on its composition. The freezing point of ice cream mixture is around −5.5°C. Lightweight sugar compounds such as glucose can cause a decrease in the freezing point of the mixture. On the other hand, the amount of frozen water in the ice cream upon exiting the freezer depends on the freezing point of the mixture. As the freezing point decreases, the amount of frozen water in the ice cream increases (Figure 12.3).

12.2.7 Ice Cream Melting Rate

The melting rate of ice cream is an important characteristic influenced by the composition of the ice cream mixture. Standard equipment for measuring the melting rate and the melting curve of ice cream is shown in Figure 12.4. The melting rate of ice cream is expressed as the percentage of weight melted

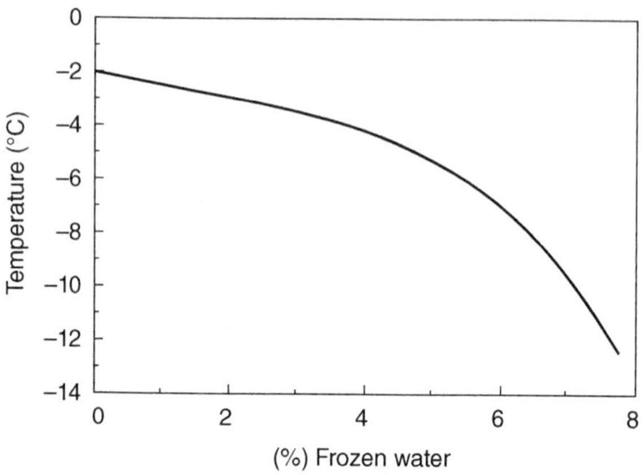

Figure 12.3 Relationship between the amount of frozen water in ice cream and freezing point.

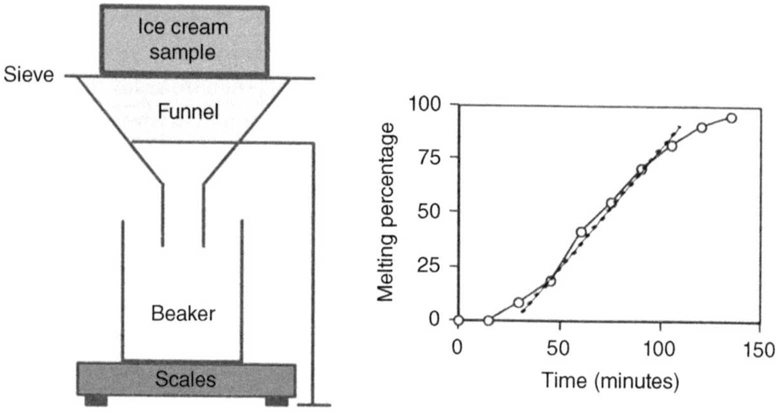

Figure 12.4 Depicts standard equipment for measuring melting speed and melting curve of ice cream.

per unit of time (minutes). A high-quality ice cream should begin melting at a satisfactory rate within 10–15 minutes at room temperature, forming a flowing and uniform liquid. The melt resistance or melt endurance test indicates how long ice cream can resist melting when exposed to high temperatures for a specific period of time. Unlike other thermal properties, melting is not a standardized physical parameter. It is essentially a laboratory measurement influenced by various factors such as thermal conductivity, heat capacity, structure, and formulation. It can be used, for example, to study the effects of formulation changes or processes on ice cream properties. In this test, a standardized ice cream container (e.g. 1 liter) is placed on a wire mesh tray inside a closed chamber at an elevated temperature (e.g. 25°C), while the initial temperature of the ice cream is lower (e.g. 18°C). Underneath the wire mesh tray, a receptacle is positioned to collect the melted ice cream. A container is placed on a balance under the receptacle to measure the weight of the melted ice cream. Additionally, by placing a graduated cylinder under the receptacle, the volume of the melted ice cream can also be measured. The weight or volume of the melted ice cream is then recorded as a percentage relative to the initial weight or volume. The resulting data is plotted as a curve against time. This test is valuable both in research and development as well as in quality control processes.

12.2.8 Aeration Capability

The aeration capability is another important feature of ice cream mixture, influenced by the composition of the mixture and the duration of mixing. As the mixing duration increases and enzymatic hydrolysis of casein proteins occurs, the aeration capability is enhanced. Essentially, aeration involves the simultaneous freezing and injection of air into the mixture. The amount of air that the mixture can retain during freezing in the freezer is referred to as the aeration capability of the mixture.

12.3 Chemical Properties

12.3.1 Gel Formation

Gel is formed as a result of the accumulation of hydrated particles. The gel has a three-dimensional structure of chains that trap free water in the spaces between the chains. These chains intersect at various points, creating a structure resembling a honeycomb. The formation of these extremely delicate chains (ultramicroscopic) is due to the alignment of particles following each other, resulting in groups of like molecules coming together side by side. The joining of these groups together causes the molecules and colloidal particles to adhere to each other, forming filaments. In some cases, especially when gel formation occurs at a relatively constant temperature, it seems that molecular rearrangement occurs again. This enhances the adhesion between particles and specific groups present in the molecules. At this point, a sol is formed and then the sol structure transforms into a gel structure. Gelatin prevents the conversion of sol to gel at this stage. Studies show that gelatin exists in the form of a sol at temperatures above 38°C. In gelatin, this temperature is referred to as the "sol-gel transition point." When gelatin solutions are cooled below this temperature, they transform into a gel, and their optical activity changes. At any temperature (below

38°C), the sol-gel equilibrium is established. With decreasing temperature, the equilibrium shifts toward the gel state. However, the rate of sol-gel conversion decreases (meaning that establishing equilibrium will take more time). The mixtures containing gelatin, which were initially tempered at around 20°C for several hours and then continued to be frozen at lower temperatures, exhibited significantly higher viscosity compared to samples frozen at lower temperatures from the start. The phenomenon was justified as follows: When a mixture is rapidly cooled, the equilibrium gel structure will be less pronounced, meaning that the gel structure present in the sol-gel equilibrium will be less developed. On the other hand, the higher the extent of gel in the sol-gel equilibrium, the more particles will connect to the gel in the form of side branches, resulting in the formation of a larger gel structure. Conversely, if the mixture is held at a high temperature (below the transition point) for a certain period, only a part of the gelatin will transform into a gel, and it will be distributed throughout the mixture. Consequently, the gelatin has not fully formed a complete gel structure (a fully three-dimensional gel structure has not formed). As the temperature is subsequently lowered, more filaments are formed and they connect with dispersed gel portions, creating an extensive gel structure. The formation of a three-dimensional and extensive gel structure increases viscosity. This phenomenon holds true for both gelatin solutions and mixtures like ice cream containing gelatin.

12.3.1.1 Gel Formation in Ice Cream

Gel formation is also possible in ice cream. Ice cream mix undergoes the process of sol-gel transformation as conditions change. The ability to form a gel structure in ice cream is due to the application of gelatin in the mixture, which depends on the amount of gelatin and its gelling strength. The gelling strength of gelatin is influenced by the amount of water in the mixture, the freezing temperature, the aging time, and the absence of agitation during the freezing process. In ice creams that use texture improvers such as enzymes (enzyme-modified ice cream), the mixture inherently displays a gel-like structure. The resulting gel-like structure can exhibit various degrees of firmness and solidity, depending on the amount of enzyme used, the acidity of the mixture, pH, temperature, enzyme activity duration, and the salts present in the mixture. This gel-like structure is related to the coagulation of caseins (similar to cheese making). The gel-like structure in frozen desserts is of significant importance, but it does not necessarily mean an increase in water hydration. The strength of the gel is due to the formation of filaments (chain-like structures) of colloidal particles that trap free liquid in capillary spaces (micelles) created within the filaments.

Creating a soft texture in ice cream through gel formation appears to be more related to the prevention of gel formation from large ice crystals. However, a portion of this property is also related to water binding to the surface of gel particles. Common gel-forming ingredients used in ice cream include stabilizers, gelatin, agar, carrageenans, and sodium alginate.

12.4 Rheological Properties

Rheology is a scientific discipline that deals with the study of material responses to applied forces. The rheological properties of food materials are crucial in process design, quality control, stability assessment during storage, process evaluation, and predicting the texture quality of products. According to the Einstein equation (Eq. (12.1)), the viscosity of an emulsion is directly affected by the continuous phase. Therefore, any alteration in the rheological properties of the continuous phase will have an impact on the overall rheology of the emulsion. The presence of thickeners in the organic phase of oil-in-water emulsions significantly influences the rheological properties of the entire system.

$$\eta = \eta_0(1 + 2.5\phi) \tag{12.1}$$

In this equation, η the viscosity of the suspension, η_0 the viscosity of the continuous phase, and ϕ the volume fraction of the dispersed phase are represented. The dispersed phase particles, due to their encapsulation by the viscoelastic membrane, exhibit a spherical state, exerting a minimal effect on the rheology of food emulsions. The apparent viscosity of the ice cream mixture increases nonlinearly by adding substances like sodium carboxymethyl cellulose, carrageenan, guar, and locust bean gum. The power model (Eq. (12.2)) is employed to study the rheological properties of the ice cream mixture.

$$\sigma = K\gamma^n \tag{12.2}$$

In this equation, σ the shear stress value (mPa) is denoted by τ, K represents the consistency coefficient (mPa·s), γ stands for the shear rate value (s^{-1}), and n is the flow behavior index.

12.4.1 Apparent and True Viscosity

Viscosity is one of the rheological properties of ice cream mixture, defined as the resistance of a fluid to flow or internal friction. Common units for expressing viscosity are millipascal seconds (mPa·s) and centipoise (cp), which are equivalent to each other. Viscosity can be categorized into two types: true viscosity (for Newtonian fluids) and apparent viscosity (for non-Newtonian fluids). The viscosity of food liquids is measured using a rotational viscometer.

Factors Affecting Fluid Viscosity Include:

1. **Temperature:** Viscosity generally decreases with an increase in temperature.
2. **Solutes' Concentration in Solution:** There is usually a nonlinear direct relationship between the concentration of solutes and the viscosity of the solution at a constant temperature.
3. **Molecular Weight of Solutes:** A nonlinear relationship often exists between the molecular weight of solutes and the viscosity of a solution at a constant concentration. An increase in molecular weight tends to increase the solution's viscosity.
4. **Pressure:** Viscosity of most liquids remains relatively constant within the range of 0–100 atmospheres of pressure. However, since food materials are not in gaseous form, the effect of pressure on their viscosity is usually disregarded.
5. **Suspension Solids' Concentration:** With an increase in the concentration of suspended solids in suspensions, viscosity dramatically increases, and the type of flow may even change. This means that non-Newtonian flow can transform into plastic or dilatant flow.

Ice cream mixture possesses both apparent viscosity (which decreases with an increase in shear rate) and true viscosity (the level of resistance the mixture maintains against flow after the disappearance of apparent viscosity). The true viscosity of the ice cream mixture ranges between 300 and 500 centipoise.

12.4.2 Determination of Rheological Properties

To determine the rheological properties of fluids, rheometers are used. Using a rheometer, controlled shear stress or shear rate is applied to the sample, and their responses are measured. Properties such as apparent viscosity or yield stress are measured based on these responses. A rheometer consists of four main components:

1. Sample location
2. Means to generate controlled shear stress or shear rate over a wide range
3. Means to measure the response
4. Means to control the temperature

It is crucial to be able to measure rheological properties over a wide range of temperatures and shear rates that ice cream experiences during

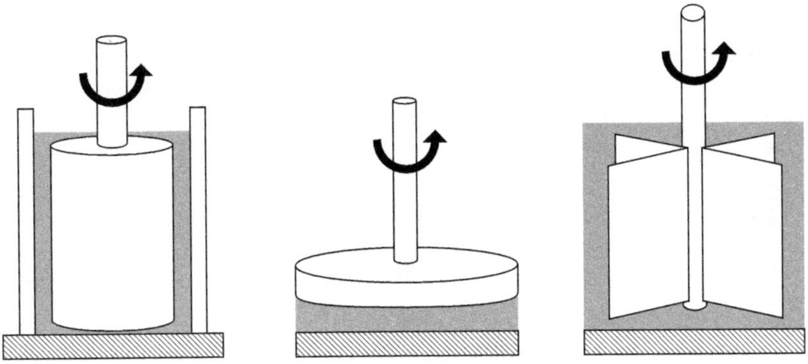

Figure 12.5 Types of rheometers – cylinder, plate, and cone.

production and distribution. In Figure 12.5, common shapes of these instruments are illustrated from a geometrical standpoint. The cylindrical shape is suitable for mixtures or melted ice cream. The cylinder rotates, and the torque is measured. The plate type is more useful at relatively higher temperatures (Figure 12.6). Pieces of ice cream (usually with a diameter of 40 mm and thickness of 4 mm) are taken and placed between the plates, equilibrating their temperature with the surroundings. For measurement, one of the plates rotates, while the other measures the torque. This type of rheometer is not suitable for ice cream at low temperatures as it becomes

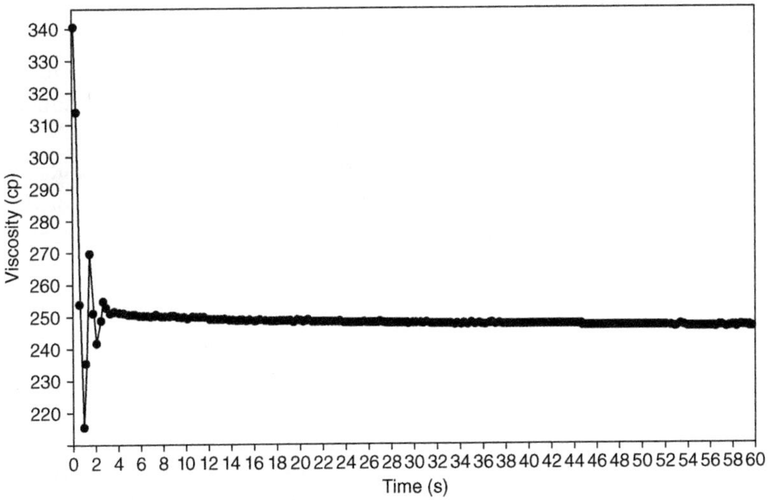

Figure 12.6 Diagram of the fungilab viscometer for low-fat ice cream. Source: Adapted from Homayouni (2008).

highly viscous, and sticks to the plate surface. For lower temperatures, the cone-and-plate type is used. The cone is immersed in a container of ice cream, and torque is applied. Above a certain threshold torque, the cone starts to rotate. The yield stress is calculated based on the dimensions of the cone and the maximum torque applied.

12.4.3 Factors Affecting the Viscosity of Ice Cream Mix

The viscosity of ice cream mix is primarily influenced by the following factors:

1. **Composition of the Mixture, Types, and Quality of Ingredients:** Among the constituent components of ice cream mix, fat, stabilizers, and salts (such as calcium, sodium, citrates, and phosphates) have the most significant impact on the viscosity of the mix. With an increase in the concentration of guar gum, apparent viscosity and storage modulus (G') also increase. Adding 0.2% guar gum, the apparent viscosity of the mix increases from 0.14 Pa.s at a shear rate of 8 rpm to 0.94 Pa.s. Additionally, reducing the fat content of the ice cream mix from 10 to 2.5% results in a decrease in apparent viscosity at a shear rate of 29.3 s^{-1} from 82.2 to 18.8 mPa.s. The effect of salts on the viscosity of ice cream mix occurs through interactions with caseins and other milk proteins.
2. **Mixture Concentration (Dry Matter Content):** It is evident that the concentration of the mixture directly affects the apparent viscosity of the mix. With an increase in dry matter content to 36.1%, the apparent viscosity increases from 0.14 to 0.6 Pa.s.
3. **Processing Type:** Significant processing methods affecting the rheological properties of ice cream mix include pasteurization, homogenization, and aging. Pasteurization, through its influence on the formation of heat-induced complexes between soluble milk proteins and caseins, affects the viscosity of the mix. One-step homogenization leads to the clustering of fat globules, thereby increasing the viscosity of the mix. During aging, due to water absorption by stabilizers and partial crystallization of milk fat, the viscosity of the mix increases.

12.4.4 Methods for Evaluating Ice Cream Mix Viscosity

The most important methods for evaluating the viscosity of ice cream mix are as follows:

1. **Measurement of Flow Time Under Constant High Pressure:** In this method, the time required for the mixture to flow under constant high-pressure capillary viscometer a specific tube or pipette is measured.

2. **Measurement of Force Required for the Movement of Parallel Plate Viscometer or Concentric Cylinder Viscometer or Concentric Plate Viscometer:** In this method, the force required to move one of two parallel plates or coaxial cylinders inside the sample is measured. In a rotational viscometer, the ice cream mixture is placed between two concentric cylinders, and the force needed to rotate the inner cylinder at a constant speed is measured.
3. **Measurement of the Fall Time of a Metal Sphere in a Column of the Mixture:** In this method, the time taken for a metal sphere to fall through a column of the ice cream mixture is measured.

12.4.5 Application of Mixture Viscosity in Freezer Design and Prediction of Final Product Quality

1. **Design of Freezing Devices:** In general, the higher the viscosity of the ice cream mixture, the greater the power required for its freezing process.
2. **Prediction of Final Product Quality:** Although numerous studies have been conducted on the factors affecting ice cream mixture viscosity and the effects of viscosity on the final product quality, the question of how much viscosity the mixture should possess and how it can be accurately determined remains a topic of discussion. For instance, proper mixing and aeration of the mixture, as well as its air retention capability, require the viscosity to be at an appropriate level. Therefore, there is a general consensus that higher viscosity in the mixture is desirable. However, for rapid freezing of the mixture using modern equipment, lower viscosity appears to be preferable. Generally, an increase in viscosity enhances resistance against melting and contributes to the smoothness and creaminess of the ice cream texture. However, the whipping speed decreases. Consequently, the viscosity of the mixture significantly impacts the texture and aerating ability of the final product. Studies indicate that gums like carob bean gum and guar gum limit the growth rate of ice crystal during recrystallization by increasing the viscosity of the mixture.

12.5 Microbial Properties of Ice Cream

Fermentation of ice cream mix leads to the production of various flavors, including tangy, fruity, cheesy, aged (moldy), and rancid flavors. Among these, tangy flavor is quite common. The tangy taste is primarily caused by lactic acid. The tangy aroma is also a result of compounds such as acetic acid, butyric acid, propionic acid, acetone, ethyl alcohol, ethyl acetate, stearaldehyde, diacetyl, and methyl ketocarbinol. Even if lactic acid is neutralized, the tangy aroma can still persist in the product due to these compounds. Therefore, ice cream with low acidity might still have a tangy aroma.

12.6 Ice Cream Microstructure

The main composition of regular ice cream consists of 17–10% milk fat, 11–8% milk solids-nonfat (lactose, proteins, and mineral salts), 17–13% sugar, 0.2–0.5% stabilizing and emulsifying mixture, and water. Water is the most important component of ice cream's composition. During the freezing of the ice cream mixture, a complex structure forms (Figure 12.7). In addition to water freezing, the incorporation of air and formation of air bubbles in ice cream are of great importance. As observed in Figure 12.6, ice crystals (b) with an average diameter of 40 microns are dispersed in the unfrozen phase, and solutes like sugars, salts, and proteins in the unfrozen phase (c) become concentrated. Air bubbles (a), with diameters around 100–40 microns, are distributed in the serum phase. The surface of these bubbles is covered by a boundary layer of serum phase containing fat globules. The volume of injected air in ice cream is approximately 50% of the total product volume.

The size of ice crystals in ice cream can be used as a criterion for evaluating its quality. If the average diameter of ice crystals is larger than 56 ± 21

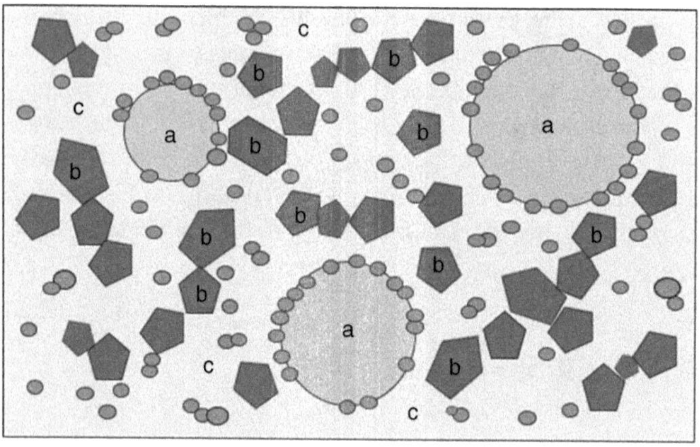

Figure 12.7 Schematic representation of ice cream microstructure after freezing: air bubbles (a), ice crystals (b), and unfrozen phase (c).

microns, the ice cream texture will be coarse. On the other hand, structural stability and the melting behavior of ice cream are important qualitative aspects. Additionally, the instability of the bottom structure contributes to the creation of an icy texture. The rheological behavior resulting from the size of air bubbles affects the mouth feel properties. Therefore, it is necessary for producers to have a comprehensive understanding of the texture formation process and the factors influencing the fine structure of ice cream (Homayouni et al. 2018).

12.6.1 Observation of Ice Cream Microstructure

For observing the microstructure of ice cream, optical or electron microscopes are used (Figure 12.8). The working method with an optical microscope is simpler, easier, and more affordable, but its resolution is limited, and to visualize the sample, the structure of the product needs to be altered or destructed. Therefore, the observed structure may differ from the actual ice cream structure. Electron microscopy offers higher magnification and precision, but it is significantly more expensive and complex. In this method, electrons are emitted from a source toward the sample and are accelerated by a positive voltage. These emitted electrons are focused on the sample using magnetic lenses and metallic equipment. Electron microscopy includes two types: scanning electron microscopy and transmission electron microscopy.

12.6.2 Determination of Fat Structure in Ice Cream

In addition to microscopic methods, there are other techniques for studying fats in ice cream. Laser diffraction is a method used to determine the size of fat globules. For this purpose, ice cream samples are dissolved in distilled

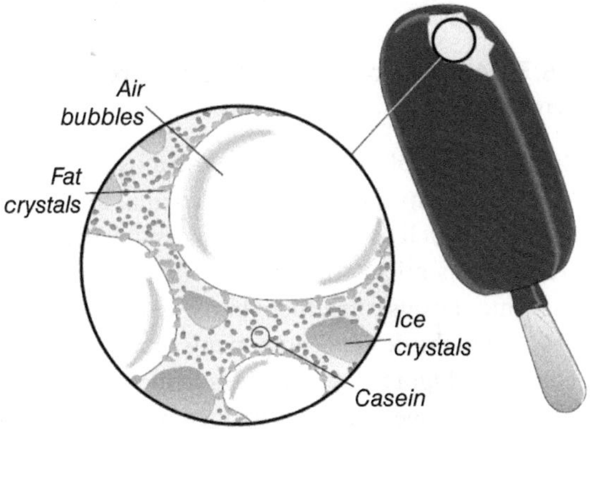

Figure 12.8 Microscopic structure of ice cream.

water, and fat globules are well separated from the solution. If necessary, a small amount of surfactant can be added to break down fat floccules, making the analysis of the diffraction pattern easier, which is used to calculate particle sizes. Quick and easy methods such as turbidity measurement and solvent extraction provide less detail compared to microscopy or light diffraction. These methods are mostly used to determine the amount of destabilized fats. In the turbidity method, they allow light to pass through a diluted solution of melted ice cream and measure the reduction in light intensity (indicating light absorption). For a fixed amount of fat, larger fat masses have fewer total surface areas compared to when the fat is in the form of fine droplets. Therefore, they scatter less light and consequently absorb less light. Comparing the light absorption of mixed ice cream (a_{mix}) with the light absorption of melted ice cream (a_{melt}) indicates the amount of destabilized fats.

$$\text{DSF}(\%) = \left(\frac{a_{\text{mix}} - a_{\text{melt}}}{a_{\text{mix}}}\right) \times 100$$

Another method involves using a solvent to separate unemulsified fats. The less emulsified the fat is, the easier it is to extract. Approximately, 10 grams of the mixture or melted ice cream and 30 milliliters of a solvent such as heptane are placed in a flask and placed in a rotary evaporator to dissolve the emulsified fats in the solvent. Then the flask is left stationary for a while to allow the solvent to separate. In the next step, the fat solution is separated from the solvent and the solvent is evaporated using heat to leave the remaining fat. The obtained fat amount, which is the fat extracted from the initial solution ($m_{extracted}$), divided by the total fat amount (m_{total}), indicates the degree of fat destabilization (DSF), which can be expressed as a percentage.

$$\text{DSF}(\%) = \left(\frac{m_{\text{extracted}}}{m_{\text{total}}}\right) \times 100$$

12.6.3 Analysis of Images Obtained from Ice Cream Microstructure

When an image of a sample is obtained using one of the microscopic methods, it can be captured, usually in a digital format on a computer. To access finer details such as the size of ice crystals, the image needs to be analyzed to examine its microstructure. The first step toward this is segmenting the image into various constituent parts. This can be done manually by drawing lines around the desired components or automatically with the assistance of a computer. Figure 12.9 illustrates a micrograph obtained from an electron microscope image of a frozen ice cream mixture. It has been divided into two

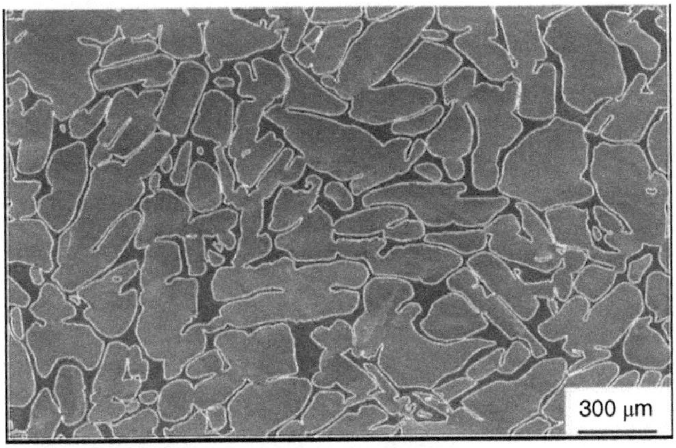

Figure 12.9 Electron microscope image of frozen ice cream with a scale bar of 300 micrometers where ice crystals are separated from the ice cream matrix using white boundary lines.

parts, ice and matrix, using white lines that are visible. By dividing an image into distinct segments, structural features, including the size of ice crystals and air bubbles, can be measured.

As shown in Figure 12.7, ice crystals and air bubbles are not perfectly spherical. Therefore, several methods can be used for their measurement and analysis. These include determining the maximum diameter, the minimum diameter, or the equivalent circle diameter (which has the same area). The shape factor, determined using the equation below, indicates the degree of sphericity of a particle. Its value is 1 for a perfect sphere, and as the shape becomes less spherical, its value decreases.

$$\text{Shape factor} = \frac{(\text{Area} \times 4\pi)}{(\text{Perimeter})^2}$$

Ice crystals and air bubbles are not all of the same size, and it is necessary to determine their size distribution in ice cream. This means figuring out what percentage of them has what size. For an accurate determination of particle size distribution, a large number of them (usually several hundred) need to be measured. Therefore, multiple images may be obtained from a single sample. Expressing the average size is generally easier. There are various methods for calculating the average, with the simplest being, to sum up, the sizes of all particles and divide by the total number of particles. However, the presence of very small particles can introduce errors in these calculations. In addition to the size and shape of ice cream structure components, their connections also have a significant impact on its physical and sensory properties. One way to measure this factor is shown in Figure 12.10.

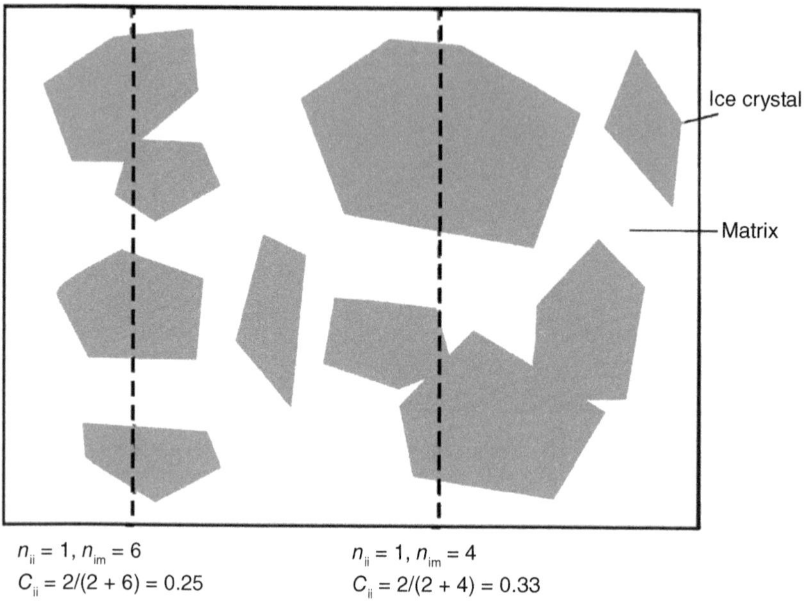

Figure 12.10 Schematic image of frozen ice cream and the method for calculating the contact factor.

In this figure, the microstructure of frozen ice cream with two phases, ice and matrix, is observed. Linear lines are drawn on the image, and the number of connections between ice and ice (n_{ii}) as well as ice and matrix (n_{im}) is counted per unit length. The value of the ice contiguity factor (C_{ii}) is calculated from the equation below. Since, in this calculation, different numbers are obtained depending on where the line is drawn in the image, several lines are usually drawn, and the average value is calculated.

$$C_{ii} = \left(\frac{2n_{ii}}{(2n_{ii} + n_{im})} \right)$$

12.7 Quality Control of Ice Cream in Practice

Quality control in ice cream production is a crucial process to ensure that the final product meets the desired standards and maintains its sensory attributes, safety, and consistency. Several methods and parameters are employed to monitor and control the quality of ice cream:

1. **Physical Tests:** Various physical tests are performed to evaluate the texture and consistency of ice cream. These tests include measuring

viscosity, hardness, melt-down resistance, and overrun (the amount of air incorporated during freezing).

2. **Chemical Analysis:** Chemical analysis is carried out to determine the composition of the ice cream, including fat content, sugar content, protein content, and moisture content. Deviations from the expected composition can impact the taste and texture of the product.
3. **Microbiological Testing:** Microbiological analysis ensures that the ice cream is free from harmful pathogens and microorganisms that could cause spoilage. This is especially important for ensuring food safety.
4. **Sensory Evaluation:** Trained sensory panels or consumer taste tests are conducted to assess the appearance, flavor, texture, and overall acceptability of the ice cream. This helps identify any deviations from the desired sensory characteristics.
5. **Quality Management Systems:** Implementing quality management systems such as good manufacturing practices (GMPs) and hazard analysis and critical control points (HACCPs) helps establish guidelines and procedures for maintaining quality and preventing contamination. By implementing these quality control measures, ice cream manufacturers can consistently produce high-quality products that meet consumer expectations and ensure food safety.

12.7.1 Physicochemical Controls

Chemical experiments of ice cream are comprehensively outlined in the standard ice cream brochure numbered 2450. In this context, only the important and practical ice cream experiments are explained in a simple manner. When we intend to conduct a test on an ice cream sample, we first record its complete specifications in a logbook. These specifications include the production date, expiration date, net weight, and packaging type. The ice cream inside the container must be filled accurately to within ±5 grams.

12.7.1.1 Measurement of Moisture and Dry Matter in Ice Cream

An empty plate is placed in an oven at 105°C for 1–0.5 hours and then cooled in a desiccator before weighing. A 5-gram sample is taken using a pipette, placed on the weighing plate, and then placed in the 105°C oven for 4–5 hours (until a constant weight is achieved). Finally, the sample is cooled in a desiccator and weighed. The percentage of moisture in the ice cream is obtained from the following formula:

$$\text{Moisture percentage} = \left(\frac{\text{Final weight of plate and sample} - \text{Initial plate weight}}{\text{Sample weight}}\right) \times 100$$

From the moisture percentage of the ice cream, we can determine its dry matter percentage:

$$\text{Dry matter percentage} = 100 - \text{Moisture percentage}$$

12.7.1.2 Measurement of Ice Cream Acidity

The ice cream is removed from freezing conditions and thoroughly mixed at laboratory temperature to achieve uniformity. Then, 3 grams of it are placed in an Erlenmeyer flask, and 20 milliliters of distilled water and a few drops of phenolphthalein are added. The mixture is gently stirred, followed by titration with 0.1 N (one-tenth normal) sodium hydroxide (NaOH) solution. The percentage of acidity is calculated using the following formula:

$$\text{Acidity percentage} = \frac{100 \times 90 \times \text{Volume of consumed sodium hydroxide solution}}{10000 \times 3(\text{Sample weight})}$$

According to food regulations, the acidity of ice cream should fall within the range of 0.08–0.18%. It is worth mentioning that the acidity of fruit-flavored ice creams, whether with or without milk, is calculated based on citric acid using the following equation:

$$\text{Percentage of acidity} = \frac{\text{Volume of consumed sodium hydroxide solution} \times 0.0064}{\text{Sample weight} \times 100}$$

12.7.1.3 Measurement of Ice Cream Overrun

The overrun of ice cream represents the percentage increase in the volume of ice cream compared to its initial volume of the mixture. For example, if we transform one liter of mixture into 1.5 liters of ice cream due to aeration, the product volume has increased by 50%. In other words, the mentioned expansion coefficient is 50%. Various methods are used to measure the overrun of ice cream, among which the weight-based method is the most commonly used. To do this, an empty ice cream cup is weighed, then it is filled with the ice cream mixture using a ladle, and the net weight of the mixture is obtained. Then, the cup is emptied and filled with ice cream taken out of the freezer. The surface of the ice cream is smoothed to the edges of the cup using a spatula, and it is weighed. The expansion coefficient of ice cream is calculated using the following formula:

$$\text{Overrun} = \frac{\text{Weight of ice cream at same volume} - \text{Weight of ice cream mixture}}{100 \times \text{Weight of ice cream at same volume}}$$

In food control laboratories, the cup filled with ice cream is weighed, melted, and poured into a graduated cylinder, and its volume is recorded. Then, the empty cup is weighed, and the net weight of ice cream is obtained. Finally, the ratio of volume to weight of ice cream is overrun. According to food regulation standards, the volume-to-weight ratio should be within the range of 2– 2.5.

12.7.1.4 Measurement of Ice Cream Fat Percentage

To measure the fat percentage in ice cream, we use a Neusal solution, which is prepared using the following method: 100 grams of trisodium citrate is dissolved in 480 milliliters of distilled water with 100 grams of sodium salicylate at mild heat. The mixture is then cooled. Next, 172 milliliters of isobutyl alcohol is added, and the volume is brought to 1.5 liters with distilled water. Finally, 0.1–0.2 grams of methylene blue powder is added. Weigh 4.42 grams of melted ice cream in ice cream butirometer, add 12 milliliters of the Neusal solution, and then close the lid of the butirometer (which should be dry) and gently shake. Gas may accumulate inside the butirometer, causing its contents to overflow. Carefully open the lid and place it in a water bath at 60°C for 5 minutes. Then, close the lid and shake. If the contents of the butirometer have not risen to the graduated tube, add a few milliliters of distilled water to make the fat level readable. Finally, place the butirometer symmetrically in a Gerber centrifuge for 10 minutes. After centrifugation, leave it in a water bath at 60°C for two minutes and then read the fat content. There is a faster method involving acid, where 10 milliliters of 90% sulfuric acid is mixed with 5 grams of ice cream and 5 milliliters of distilled water along with 1–2 milliliters of isoamyl alcohol in a Gerber butirometer. This mixture is centrifuged for 5 minutes, and then the fat is read from the butirometer.

12.7.1.5 Identification of the Type of Fat Used in Ice Cream

A portion of extracted fat is melted and filtered using regular filter paper. 5 grams of it are taken and weighed in a 300-milliliter distillation flask (Figure 12.11). 20 milliliters of sodium glycerol solution are added to it, and the mixture is heated until it becomes completely clear. Then, 135 milliliters of freshly boiled distilled water are gradually added. After that, 6 milliliters of sulfuric acid are added drop by drop. Several boiling stones are also added to prevent bumping inside the flask. By connecting the flask to the distillation apparatus and placing it on a noncombustible plate, distillation is carried out. The flame is adjusted in a way that around 110 milliliters of the distillation product are collected in 30 minutes. After approximately 110 milliliters have been collected, the flame is turned off, and instead of the receiving container, a 25 milliliter graduated cylinder is placed under the

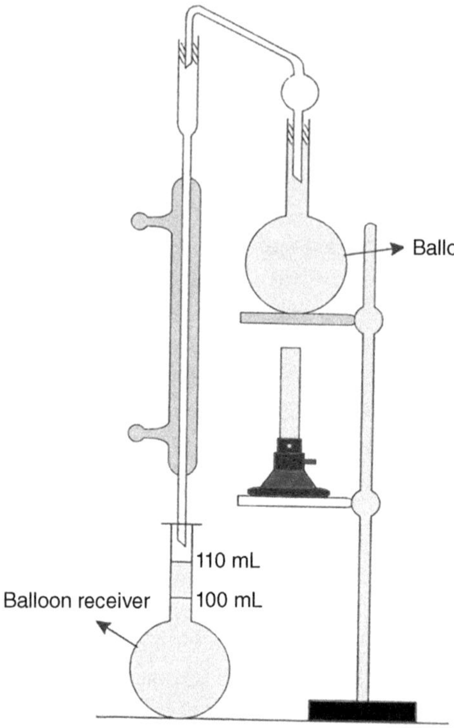

Figure 12.11 A schematic of the distillation apparatus by Reichert-Meissl.

apparatus to collect any remaining drops that might condense after turning off the flame. The receiving container is gently shaken to mix its contents. Then, the container is immersed in water at 15°C for 15 minutes, and the contents are filtered dry using a regular filter paper with a diameter of 90 milliliters. Next, 100 milliliters of the filtered substance are titrated with a 0.1 N NaOH standard solution, using 0.5 milliliters of a 0.5% phenolphthalein indicator until a pink color appears. Titration is complete when the pink color remains stable for 2–3 minutes.

Control Test: This test is carried out similarly to the previous method, using equal amounts of substances, but instead of the test sample, distilled water is used.

Calculation Method: Based on the following formula, we calculate the Reichert-Meissl value.

$$\text{Reichert-Meissl value} = (\text{Volume used in the titration for control} - \text{Volume used in the titration for sample}) \times \frac{1}{1}$$

The Reichert-Meissl value for animal oil or butter is 32–24. The Reichert-Meissl value for vegetable butter (margarine) is a maximum of 2. Values between these two numbers indicate a mixture of both types of oil.

12.7.1.6 Sucrose Percentage Measurement

Weigh two grams of ice cream sample in a beaker (100 milliliters) and dissolve it in distilled water. Transfer the solution to a volumetric flask (100 milliliters), adjust the volume, and filter if necessary.

Take 25 milliliters of the obtained solution and transfer it to another volumetric flask, then add enough water to reach the desired volume and pour it into a burette.

Mix 5 milliliters of Fehling A solution and 5 milliliters of Fehling B solution in a flask, heat on a heater until boiling, and titrate with the sugar solution in the presence of Benedict's reagent. Continue titration until the solution becomes colorless and a reddish cuprous oxide precipitate forms. Use the following formula to calculate the percentage of sugar before hydrolysis:

$$\text{Percentage of sugar before hydrolysis} = \frac{(100 \times 100 \times 100 \times \text{Fehling factor})}{(1000 \times 25 \times \text{Sample weight}(2\text{ grams}) \times \text{Volume used})}$$

Then, take another 25 milliliters of the initial 2% solution, pour it into a volumetric flask (100 milliliters), add 5 milliliters of concentrated hydrochloric acid, and heat it at 70°C for 10 minutes. Cool the sample afterward. In the presence of resorcinol, observe the development of a pale pink color (onion skin color). Neutralize with 20% hydrochloric acid if needed, adjust the volume, and pour it into a burette. Mix 5 milliliters of Fehling A solution and 5 milliliters of Fehling B solution in a flask containing some distilled water and boiling stones. Titrate while boiling. Use the following formula to calculate the percentage of sugar after hydrolysis:

$$\text{Percentage of sugar after hydrolysis} = \frac{(100 \times 100 \times 100 \times \text{Fehling factor})}{(1000 \times 25 \times \text{Sample weight (2 grams)} \times \text{Volume used})}$$

Calculate the percentage of sucrose using the equation:

$$\text{Sucrose percentage} = \left(\text{Sugar percentage before hydrolysis} - \text{Sugar percentage after hydrolysis}\right) \times 0.95$$

12.7.1.7 Measurement of MSNF in Ice Cream

Transfer 10 grams of the prepared ice cream sample to an Erlenmeyer flask. Add 1 milliliter of phenolphthalein solution to it and neutralize its acidity with 0.1 normal NaOH solution. Then, add 3 milliliters of formalin to the sample and neutralize it once again to develop a pink color using 0.1 normal NaOH solution. Let us denote the volume of NaOH solution consumed as "X" milliliters. In addition, take 3 milliliters of formalin and neutralize it in the presence of phenolphthalein using 0.1 normal NaOH solution. Denote the volume of NaOH solution consumed as "Y" milliliters. Using the following formula, calculate the percentage of nonfat solid content (MSNF) in the ice cream:

$$\text{MSNF percentage in ice cream} = ((X - Y) \times 5.67)$$

12.7.2 Microbiological Controls

The microbial content of ice cream primarily reflects the quality of the ingredients used in its production, including raw milk, MSNF, cream, sugar, fruits, chocolate, eggs, stabilizers, and emulsifiers. Raw milk and its soluble components are typically combined and subjected to pasteurization. As a result, microbial counts in the pasteurized blend are usually low, often below 100 mL^{-1}. Bacillus species and some thermoduric bacteria are usually the only survivors after pasteurization. However, contamination can occur during the addition of coloring agents, flavors, and other components, such as chocolate, fruits, and nuts, after pasteurization. Furthermore, post-pasteurization contamination can result from factors such as air and water mixtures, inadequately cleaned equipment, personal items, improper use of product remnants, and the use of unsanitary and contaminated packaging materials. The presence of coliform bacteria in pasteurized ice cream is an indication of post-pasteurization contamination. Ice cream has also been associated with the transmission of pathogens such as *Escherichia coli (E. coli)*, *Listeria*, *Salmonella*, *Campylobacter*, *Yersinia*, and *Staphylococcus*, which are significant causes of foodborne illnesses in humans. Recommended microbiological methods for assessing the quality of ice cream include the following parameters:

1. Standard Plate Count (SPC)
2. Enterobacteriaceae Count
3. Coliform Count
4. Thermoduric Count
5. Psychrotrophic Count
6. *Staphylococcus aureus* Count
7. Yeast-Mold Count

The results of these microbial examinations are typically expressed as the number of microorganisms per gram of ice cream. According to international standards, the acceptable limits for the number of live microorganisms per gram of ice cream are as follows:

- **Total Count or Total Aerobic Mesophilic Bacterial Count:** Should not exceed 10^5.
- **Enterobacteriaceae:** Should not exceed 10^2.
- ***Staphylococcus aureus*:** Should not exceed 10^2.
- ***E. coli*:** Should be absent (zero) per gram of ice cream.

Additionally, it is essential to assess all bulk components before their use in the ice cream manufacturing process to ensure the quality and safety of the final product. In addition to conventional methods such as culture, microscopic examination, and sampling techniques, microbiological analysis of ice cream benefits from a range of fast and efficient techniques in various categories. These include:

Chemical Methods: These methods involve the use of chemical indicators and compounds for analysis. Examples include thermostable nuclease, radiometry, and the use of chromogenic and fluorogenic substrates.

Physical Methods: Physical techniques involve measurements of physical properties. Some relevant methods include microcalorimetry, which measures heat changes in microbial growth, and flow cytometry, a technique for counting and characterizing cells or particles in a fluid.

Immunological Methods: Immunological techniques utilize the immune system's responses for analysis. These methods include fluorescent antibody assays, enrichment serology, and ELISA (enzyme-linked immunosorbent assay).

Molecular Methods: Molecular techniques involve the analysis of genetic material, such as DNA and RNA. Examples include PCR (polymerase chain reaction) and real-time PCR, which allow for the detection and quantification of specific genetic sequences.

Chemical, physical, molecular, and immunological techniques represent newer and faster methods with high levels of accuracy and sensitivity. However, each method may have its limitations and potential shortcomings. Therefore, it is often recommended to use a combination of these methods to obtain a comprehensive and accurate assessment of the mentioned bacteria in ice cream and other dairy products. This multimethod approach helps ensure the safety and quality of the final product.

12.7.2.1 Preparation of Various Dilutions from Solid and Liquid Food Materials

In solid food materials, the first dilution, namely 0.1, is prepared as follows: Weigh 5 grams of the substance. Add 45 milliliters of physiological serum

(8.5 grams of pure table salt in 100 milliliters of distilled water) to it and mix thoroughly. Allow the mixture to stand for half an hour until the food material is completely dissolved and all liquid parts are uniformly mixed. Then, take 1 milliliter from 0.1 dilution and add to 9 milliliters of physiological serum to achieve a 0.01 dilution, and similarly prepare the other dilutions. In liquid food materials such as beverages, yoghurt, and milk, which can be drawn using a pipette, we introduce 1 milliliter of the food material itself, creating zero dilution. The remaining dilutions are prepared similarly to solid food materials by adding physiological serum. However, there is a slight difference in dilution method for culturing *Salmonella*. In this case, we pour 25 grams of the food material into a sterile glass containing 225 milliliters of lactose-bile solution. We mix it using a sterile mixer and allow it to sit for half an hour. Then, we incubate the mixture in an incubator at 37°C for 24 hours to allow the present microbes to grow. Microbes of significant importance in ice cream include aerobic microorganisms, coliform bacteria, *E. coli*, Salmonella, *Staphylococcus aureus* (Staph), molds, and yeasts.

12.7.2.2 Enumeration of Aerobic Bacteria

For the enumeration of aerobic bacteria, we use the culture medium MPH-Agar. Following the instructions provided on the label, the culture medium is prepared. Then, dilution 5 (0.00001) is prepared from the melted ice cream sample, and the poor-plate method is used for cultivation. Iñ the poor-plate method, a sample is first poured onto an empty plate. Then, the culture medium is added in two steps. The procedure is as follows: One milliliter of dilution 5 is precisely measured using a 1-milliliter pipette and poured onto a sterile plate. A quantity of culture medium (liquid) is added to cover the plate's surface. The plate is gently rotated to ensure uniform distribution. Subsequently, another quantity of the culture medium is added, allowing it to gel. Finally, the plates are inverted and incubated at 37°C in an incubator for 48 hours. After two days, the plates are placed in a colony counter device, and the number of circular-shaped, milk-colored colonies is counted. Ideally, the number of colonies on each plate should exceed 5. This is because the acceptable standard for total aerobic count is 500,000 microbes per gram (milliliter) of ice cream.

12.7.2.3 Enumeration of Coliform Bacteria

For the enumeration of coliform bacteria, the Mac Conkey Agar (MCA) culture medium is used. First, the culture medium is prepared according to the recommendations on its label. Then, from the melted ice cream under sterile conditions and at the laboratory temperature, we prepare a dilution two. The culture is performed using the poor-plate method. One milliliter of dilution two is poured onto a plate (the culture process is always performed near a flame). Then, a quantity of the culture medium is added, and the plate is gently swirled in an 8-figure motion to ensure even distribution. After that, an equal amount of culture medium is added and the plates are incubated at 37°C for 24 hours in an incubator. The next day, we examine the plates under a colony counter light. Any colonies, if present, appear as pink (the same color as the culture medium) and have a circular shape. According to the standard, dilution two should not contain any visible colonies. To ensure accurate and precise culturing, it is advisable to use other dilutions alongside the primary dilution, perform two or three replicates for each culture, and compare the results.

12.7.2.4 Enumeration of *E. coli*

For the enumeration of *E. coli*, the Brilliant Green (BG) Bile culture medium is used. The culture medium is prepared according to the manufacturer's instructions. In each test tube, a Durham tube is placed upside down, and 9 milliliters of the culture medium are added and then sterilized in an autoclave. The ice cream sample is melted beside a flame, and 1 milliliter of the ice cream itself or 10 milliliters of dilution 0.1 is taken and added to the test tube containing the culture medium. The test tube is then placed in an incubator at 37°C for 48 hours. After two days, the test tube is examined. If gas has accumulated in the Durham tube, the sample is suspicious, indicating the possible presence of *E. coli* in the sample. In this case, the test should be continued. To do this, a few drops from the mentioned test tube are added to the BG Bile medium, and a few drops are added to another test tube containing peptone water culture medium. Both tubes are placed in a water bath filled with water for 48 hours at 44°C. After two days, if no gas is formed in the BG tube, there is no contamination. However, if gas is produced again in the BG tube, three or four drops of Kovac's reagent are added to the peptone water tube. If no color change is observed, the sample is not contaminated with *E. coli*. But if a purple ring of indole forms at the top of the tube, the sample is contaminated with *E. coli*. Generally, *E. coli* should be negative in dilution zero and 0.1.

12.7.2.5 Enumeration of *Staphylococcus* (*Staph*)

For the enumeration of *Staphylococcus*, the Brilliant Parker (BP) culture medium is used. The culture medium is prepared according to the instructions on the label, and a dilution 0.1 is prepared from the ice cream. One milliliter of dilution 0.1 is poured onto a plate containing BP, and the plate is incubated at 37°C for 48–72 hours. After this period, the plate is examined under a colony counter light. If black colonies with an oily halo (resembling bubbles around the colonies) are observed, the colonies are counted and multiplied by the dilution factor. Ideally, no colonies should be observed. In food and pharmaceutical products, where the presence of *Staphylococcus* should be negative in 1 gram of sample (such as ice cream, instant soup, and paper towels), a dilution 0.1 is prepared. Ten milliliters of this dilution are added to a salted cooked-meat culture medium, and it is incubated at 37°C for 24 hours. The next day, a few drops of the previous culture medium are inoculated onto a BP culture medium, and the plate is incubated at 37°C for 48–72 hours. If black colonies with an oily halo form on the BP culture medium, then for confirming *Staphylococcus aureus*, a small amount of rabbit plasma powder is mixed with two milliliters of sterile distilled water, and then 0.5 milliliters of rabbit-plasma solution are added to a small sterile test tube. Suspicious colonies are transferred to the plasma medium using a sterile loop and mixed. If agglutination (clumping) occurs in the plasma, it confirms the presence of *Staphylococcus aureus*. If no agglutination occurs, the tube is incubated at 37°C for 24 hours. After 24 hours, if agglutination occurs, it confirms the positive presence of *Staphylococcus aureus*, otherwise *Staph* is not present in the food.

12.7.2.6 Enumeration of Mold and Yeast

For the enumeration of mold and yeast, the sabouraud dextrose agar (SBA) culture medium is used. One milliliter of dilution 0.1 is surface-inoculated onto the culture medium and incubated at 27°C for 5 days. The plates are directly placed in the incubator for 24 hours and then inverted for the remaining 4 days. After 5 days, the plates are examined under a colony counter, and the colonies are counted. Mold colonies appear as filamentous structures with visible color centers, while yeast colonies are smaller and less noticeable compared to mold colonies. Generally, the colony count should not exceed 5 colonies. Up to 50 mold and yeast colonies per gram of ice cream sample are permissible, and above that, it is reported as "contaminated."

12.7.2.7 Enumeration of Salmonella

The enumeration of *Salmonella* involves multiple stages, consisting of 5 consecutive days of culturing. Salmonella is often problematic in protein-containing foods. On the first day, 25 grams of the food sample are diluted in 225 milliliters of lactose broth enrichment medium, and the mixture is homogenized using a sterile glass rod. Then, it is incubated at 37°C for 24 hours. All equipment used must be sterile, and all steps should be performed near a flame. On the second day, 1 milliliter of the lactose broth is taken and added to selenite broth and another 1 milliliter to tetrathionate broth. Tetrathionate broth is prepared beforehand and contains 0.2 milliliters of iodine solution (potassium iodide solution) added before the sample. Tetrathionate broth is incubated at 44°C, and selenite broth is incubated at 37°C for 24 hours. On the third day, plates are divided into halves using a marker. A loopful of the previous cultures (selenite and tetrathionate) is taken with a sterile loop and zigzag streaked on new plates. Half of the plates receive selenite broth, and the other half receive tetrathionate broth. These plates are then incubated at 37°C for 24 hours. On the fourth day, the plates are examined. If no colonies are seen on both plates, *Salmonella* is negative. If colonies that are small, transparent, and rarely produce black gas (SH2) are observed in the SSA medium, the sample is suspicious. If pink colonies are observed in the BGA medium, it is a positive *Salmonella* result. If no colonies are seen in any of the media, the sample is *Salmonella* negative and the test is halted. In cases of suspicion, the test should be continued. The continuation involves streaking suspicious colonies onto TSI slants for further biochemical testing. On the fifth day, TSI slants are examined. If the bottom of the TSI slant turns yellow and the top turns purple, with a black color (SH2) and the lysine agar also turns purple, *Salmonella* is positive. Suspicious colonies are transferred to "motility," "urea," and "peptone water" culture media and incubated at 37°C for 24 hours. On the sixth day, the culture media are examined. If the urea medium does not change color, peptone water does not produce a red color (plum), and the motility medium turns cloudy, the sample is suspected to be positive for *Salmonella*. At this stage, all three culture media must confirm each other. If confirmed, the presence of *Salmonella* is verified using specific antisera on slide agglutination.

12.7.2.8 Quantifying Probiotic Microorganisms in Probiotic Ice Cream

The composition of the ice cream matrix makes it a promising carrier for probiotics. This is due to its structure, which includes milk proteins, fat, lactose, and various other components. While ice cream's composition and near-neutral pH (around 6.5) make it seem like a suitable medium for probiotic cultures, the freezing process can potentially impact their survival (Homayouni 2009; Homayouni et al. 2012). To accurately assess the viability of probiotic microorganisms, it is crucial to have a reliable method for selectively counting them. The viability of probiotics is essential for delivering their health benefits. Several strategies can enhance the survivability of probiotics, such as selecting strains that are resistant to acid and bile, using oxygen-impermeable packaging, microencapsulation, adapting probiotics to stress conditions, and incorporating micronutrients like amino acids and peptides. To provide health benefits, the recommended concentration of probiotic microorganisms in ice cream is typically 10^7 colony-forming units per gram (CFU/g). Various media have been proposed for selectively enumerating Bifidobacterium spp. and Lactobacilli in ice cream and other dairy products, including MRS-bile agar, MRS-salicin agar, MRS-sorbitol agar, MRS-maltose agar, MRS-glucose-vancomycin-agar, MRS-LP agar, MRS-IM agar, RCPB agar, DP agar, BIM-25 agar, AMC agar, MBG agar, BL-OG agar, TPPY-E agar, TOS-NNLP agar, and more. Based on the findings of most previous studies, MRS agar, equipped with selective and differential agents, is highly suitable for selectively and differentially enumerating probiotics in ice cream and various other probiotic dairy products.

References

Homayouni, A. (2008). Effect of microencapsulation and resistant starch on the probiotic survival and sensory properties of synbiotic ice cream. PhD thesis. University of Tehran, Iran.

Homayouni, A. (2009). *Therapeutical Effects of Functional Probiotic, Prebiotic and Synbiotic Foods*. Tabriz, Iran: Tabriz University of Medical Sciences.

Homayouni, A., Azizi, A., Ehsani, M.R., and Yarmand, M.S. (2008). Effect of microencapsulation and resistant starch on the probiotic survival and sensory properties of synbiotic ice cream. *Food Chemistry* 111 (1): 50–55.

Homayouni, A., Azizi, A., Javadi, M. et al. (2012). Factors influencing probiotic survival in ice cream a review. *International Journal of Dairy Science* 7 (1): 1–10.

Homayouni, A., Javadi, M., Ansari, F. et al. (2018). Advanced methods in ice cream analysis, a review. *Food Analytical Methods* 11: 3224–3234.

13

Sensory Properties of Probiotic Ice Cream

13.1 Sensory Evaluation of Ice Cream

Sensory evaluation of ice cream holds special significance. It has been proven through experience that two food items with the same composition can have different levels of acceptance among consumers. The reason a consumer prefers one of these two food items over the other originates from unfamiliar compounds that determine the characteristics of that food item. Sensory evaluation of food materials refers to methods in which instead of measurement devices and tools, the human's five senses are used to determine the level of food acceptance by consumers. These methods are also called organoleptic or sensory methods. Organ refers to "sense" and leptic comes from the word leptikos, meaning "acceptable." When an individual consumes a food item, they employ all their senses (sight, touch, smell, taste, and hearing) to perceive its attributes. For instance, the sound produced while chewing potato chips is one of the characteristics of this product and is perceived through the sense of hearing. Quality assessment tools for food materials are developed based on the performance of the human's five senses. For example, in the Proctor penetrometer, five artificial teeth are embedded, capable of performing cutting and crushing movements on the product. Based on this, the physical resistance of the food material is evaluated. In general, using human senses can provide a somewhat qualitative assessment of food quality, but this assessment is mostly comparative in nature. Human senses are only capable of detecting the intensity, weakness, and good or bad sensory attributes, and they cannot accurately determine the exact limits of these attributes. On the other hand, employing human senses for food evaluation has its limitations. The sensitivity of human senses depends on factors such as ethnicity, individual differences, physiology, age, gender, disease conditions, cold, heat, light,

Probiotic Ice Cream: Science and Technology, First Edition. Aziz Homayouni-Rad.

pressure, culture, and religion, as well as dietary preferences and smoking habits. Sensory evaluation is utilized when:

A. Physical, chemical, and biological evaluations alone are not sufficient.
B. Descriptive attributes are the subject of evaluation.
C. Quantitative attributes cannot be measured using available tools.
D. The goal is to identify factors influencing product acceptance.

Sensory properties refer to characteristics of food that are perceived through the senses of sight, smell, taste, touch, and hearing. These properties include attributes such as flavor, texture, and appearance. Taste is a combination of aroma (volatile compounds detected by the nose) and taste (sensations perceived by the tongue due to nonvolatile solids and liquids). Aroma is detected through the olfactory nerve, which extends to the upper parts of the nasal passages. The quantity of these compounds is very small, usually in the milligram per kilogram range of food. To appreciate the importance of aroma, simply pinch your nose while eating and you will notice that the food becomes tasteless. The number of volatile compounds contributing to a specific taste can be quite extensive. For instance, vanilla, strawberry, and cocoa aromas may contain between 100 and 500 different volatile compounds. Most adults can distinguish between around 2000 different aromas. These compounds are usually present in concentrations about a thousand times lower than the compounds responsible for creating the aroma. They are only distinguishable when in solution and in contact with taste receptors on the tongue. Solid substances need to be dissolved in saliva before they can be sensed. Taste buds are sensitive to five main tastes, including bitterness (caffeine and quinine), saltiness (salt), sourness (citric acid), sweetness (sugar), and umami (monosodium glutamate). Beyond the compounds that create aroma and taste, there are two other categories of molecules that affect flavor perception. These are molecules that act on trigeminal receptors, responsible for sensations of coolness, pungency (mustard and pepper), and warmth (capsaicin). Enhancers and suppressors of taste are used at low concentrations to enhance or suppress other tastes. Examples include maltol and ethyl maltol, which have a caramel-like flavor and increase the perception of sweetness. Furaneol is used to enhance the taste of red fruits or wild fruits. Vanilla can soften the bitterness of chocolate and certain fruits, as well as enhance sweetness. Sucrose can reduce bitterness, sourness, and saltiness (e.g. in chocolate) while increasing the perception of fruit flavors. It is worth noting that flavor perception is temperature-dependent, and flavors are less intense at lower temperatures. This is why more flavorful compounds are added to ice cream compared to products consumed at higher temperatures (e.g. beverages). Texture perception is derived from signals from pressure receptors in the tongue, mouth, and throat, as well as muscle receptors based on force and displacement. Texture perception is not only influenced by the properties of the product but also by the way it breaks down in the mouth. There are two main methods used to assess the sensory properties of ice cream. One involves analytical methods where trained individuals provide expert opinions, and the other involves consumer opinions gathered through questionnaires provided to them (Homayouni 2013).

13.1.1 Sensory Evaluation of Probiotic Ice Cream

The sensory evaluations of the synbiotic ice cream samples are detailed in Table 13.1. The scores assigned for attributes such as color, body texture, and taste indicate that the introduction of both free and encapsulated probiotics had no discernible impact on the sensory characteristics of the nonfermented synbiotic ice cream. None of the samples exhibited a yogurt or probiotic flavor, mainly due to the elevated pH of the nonfermented ice cream. Overall, when considering color, texture, and taste, all samples received favorable ratings and did not exhibit any noticeable off-flavors throughout the storage period. Furthermore, none of the ice creams was assessed as being crumbly, weak, fluffy, or sandy in texture.

Table 13.1 Sensory properties of synbiotic ice cream (Homayouni et al. 2008)/ with permission of Elsevier.

Samples	Color and appearance*	Body and texture	Flavor and taste	Total acceptability
	(1–5)	(1–5)	(1–10)	(1–20)
A	$4.45 \pm 0.07^{a)}$	$4.53 \pm 0.02^{a, b)}$	$9.15 \pm 0.02^{a)}$	$18.13 \pm 0.04^{a)}$
B	$4.40 \pm 0.04^{a, b)}$	$4.55 \pm 0.01^{a)}$	$9.10 \pm 0.05^{a, b)}$	$18.05 \pm 0.03^{a, b)}$
C	$4.42 \pm 0.03^{a, b)}$	$4.56 \pm 0.04^{a)}$	$9.13 \pm 0.03^{a)}$	$18.11 \pm 0.03^{a)}$
D	$4.43 \pm 0.02^{a, b)}$	$4.56 \pm 0.05^{a)}$	$9.12 \pm 0.04^{a)}$	$18.11 \pm 0.04^{a)}$
E	$4.40 \pm 0.03^{a, b)}$	$4.54 \pm 0.04^{a)}$	$9.14 \pm 0.03^{a)}$	$18.08 \pm 0.03^{a, b)}$

a, b) Means in the same column followed by different letters were significantly different ($P < 0.05$).

A: Prebiotic ice cream with free *L.casei,* B: prebiotic ice cream with encapsulated *L. casei* C: prebiotic ice cream with free *B. lactis,* D: prebiotic ice cream with encapsulated *B. lactis*, E: prebiotic ice cream with without probiotic (control).

* Mean values from 32 panelists.

13.1.2 Sensory Properties of Probiotic Ice Cream

Probiotic ice cream offers an opportunity to create distinct flavor profiles compared to traditional ice cream. Ingredients like inulin and oligofructose can enhance the sensory properties of ice cream, providing a rounder mouth feel, sustaining flavor with reduced aftertaste, and imparting a mild sweetness. These sensory attributes contribute to higher ratings for taste, creaminess, and overall acceptability of synbiotic ice cream. Flavor is a primary factor influencing food choices, followed by considerations related to health benefits. If functional ingredients introduced into ice cream impart unpleasant flavors, consumers may not be inclined to consume functional probiotic ice cream, even if it offers health advantages. Therefore, effective communication of the health benefits associated with probiotics is crucial in promoting the acceptance of functional probiotic ice cream over traditional varieties. Making these health benefits understandable to all consumers is a key aspect of developing new probiotic ice cream. While the overall acceptability of nonfermented probiotic ice cream is similar to conventional ice cream, fermented probiotic ice cream and frozen desserts with low pH values (ranging from 4.0 to 4.5) can face challenges in terms of sensory acceptance. This is because ice cream is not typically characterized as an acidic food product. However, increasing the sugar concentration can help improve sensory properties, although the addition of inulin may not have the same effect. It is noteworthy that the incorporation of specific probiotic strains, such as *L. paracasei subsp. paracasei*, and the use of inulin have been shown to positively impact sensory preferences, even in the case of mousse-based products (Homayouni et al. 2008). Balancing the sensory aspects with the health benefits is a critical consideration in the development of probiotic ice cream to ensure consumer acceptance and satisfaction.

13.2 Examination of Various Aspects of Ice Cream Quality

Any food product introduced to the market must possess high acceptability and palatability. The acceptability of a food product relies on its physical, chemical, and microbiological quality. When multiple samples of a food product are comparable in terms of physical, chemical, and microbiological attributes, their organoleptic (sensory) quality becomes the basis for comparison. In the ice cream industry as well, sensory evaluation (organoleptic) is employed for assessing and comparing product quality, using panels of experts. A panel group consists of trained individuals capable of identifying

Table 13.2 Scoring system for sensory parameters of ice cream.

Parameter	Points
Taste	10
Texture and structure	5
Color, appearance, and packaging	5
Melting quality	3
Microbial load	2
Total	25

product defects and being aware of factors causing such defects and their prevention methods. The quality and excellence of ice cream depend on its taste, texture, structure, color, appearance, packaging, melting quality, and microbial load. The American Dairy Science Association in 1987 published Table 13.2 detailing how to score sensory parameters of ice cream.

An ideal ice cream is one that has a distinct, fresh, delightful, and delicious taste, with a cohesive and soft texture. Its structure should be balanced and desirable, relatively dense, and chewable to a certain extent. It should melt gradually toward a liquid state while maintaining the appearance of the initial mixture. It should be appetizing in appearance, with natural color, and attractive packaging. Moreover, from a microbiological perspective, it should be safe and healthy. To achieve this, all components of the ice cream must be of high quality and well-mixed with specific ratios. They should be processed under proper conditions and then stored and distributed appropriately. The scoring format for evaluating various sensory parameters of ice cream is presented in Figure 13.1.

13.2.1 Taste

According to the quality scoring system previously provided, taste is the most influential factor in ice cream quality and accounts for approximately half of the overall quality value (10 points out of the total 25 points). Taste encompasses both flavor and aroma. The interaction between taste compounds and taste and smell receptors triggers a neural signal, which is immediately transmitted to the central nervous system. In the brain, the neural signal is analyzed, and the perceived taste is compared not only to the current flavor but also to the memory of previous tastes. Therefore, maintaining flavor consistency across different time periods is crucial. Other factors, such as texture and color, also impact the taste of a food item.

ICE CREAM SCORE CARD

PRODUCT: ____________________ DATE: ____________________

FLAVOR: ____________________

SAMPLE NO.

	CRITICISM	1	2	3	4	5	6	7	8	9	10
FLAVOR 10	SCORE ▶										
NO CRITICISM = 10	**FLAVORING SYSTEM** LACKS FINE FLAVOR										
	LACKS FLAVORING										
UNSALABLE = 0	TOO HIGH FLAVOR										
	UNNATURAL FLAVOR										
NORMAL RANGE = 1 10	**SWEETENERS** LACKS SWEETNESS										
	TOO SWEET										
	SYRUP FLAVOR										
	PROCESSING COOKED										
	DAIRY INGREDIENTS ACID										
	SALTY										
	LACKS FRESHNESS										
	OLD INGREDIENT										
	OXIDIZED										
	METALLIC										
	RANCID										
	WHEY										
	OTHERS STORAGE (ABSORBED)										
	STABILIZER/EMULSIFIER										
	NEUTRALIZER										
	FOREIGN										
BODY & TEXTURE 5	SCORE ▶										
NO CRITICISM = 10	COARSE/ICY										
	CRUMBLY										
	FLUFFY										
UNSALABLE = 0	GUMMY										
	SANDY										
NORMAL RANGE = 1–5	SOGGY										
	WEAK										
COLOR, APPEARANCE & PACKAGE 5	SCORE ▶										
NO CRITICISM = 5	DULL COLOR										
	NON-UNIFORM COLOR										
	TOO HIGH COLOR										
UNSALABLE = 0	TOO PALE COLOR										
	UNNATURAL COLOR										
NORMAL RANGE = 1–5	DAMAGED CONTAINER										
	DEFECTIVE SEAL										
	ILL-SHAPED CONTAINER										
	SOILED CONTAINER (DIRT)										
	SOILED CONTAINER (PRODUCT)										
	UNDER FILLED										
	OVER FILLED										
MULTING QUALITY 3	SCORE ▶										
NO CRITICISM = 3	CURDY										
	DOES NOT MELT										
UNSALABLE = 0	FLAKY										
	FOAMY										
NORMAL RANGE = 1–3	WATERY										
	WHEYED OFF										
BACTERIAL CONTENT 2	SCORE ▶										
	STANDARD PLATE COUNT										
	COLIFORM COUNT										
TOTAL 25	**TOTAL SCORE OF EACH SAMPLE**										
	TOTAL SOLIDS (%)										
	FAT CONTENT (%)										
	NET WEIGHT (LBS/GAL)										
	OVERRUN (%)										

SIGNATURE OF EVALUATORS: ____________________ ____________________ ____________________

Figure 13.1 Ice cream scorecard (Marshall et al. 2003) / with permission of Springer Nature.

For instance, the color orange in a food product can evoke the memory of an orange flavor for the consumer. If two samples of ice cream, one with a smooth texture and the other with a coarser texture, are evaluated by a panel group, the sample with a better texture will receive a higher score for taste. Excessive consumption of sugar and flavoring agents significantly affects ice cream taste. Flavoring agents must be uniformly distributed within the mixture, without being overwhelmed by the taste of other components. For example, to achieve a vanilla flavor, the ice cream should have a pleasant sweetness. Excessive or insufficient sweetness can diminish the enjoyable vanilla taste. Flavor defects in ice cream are categorized based on their causes and origins as follows:

1. **Taste defects arising from raw materials:**
   a. **Flavoring agents:** Lack of flavor, imbalanced flavor, excessive flavor, and unnatural flavor.
   b. **Sweeteners:** Lack of sweetness, excessive sweetness, and malt-like taste.
   c. **Dairy products:** Sour taste, cooked or eggy taste, rancid or aged taste, oxidized or metallic taste, curdled or overly sharp taste, salty taste, and whey taste.
   d. **Other raw materials:** Possible tastes derived from eggs, preservatives, and emulsifiers.
2. **Taste defects arising from chemical changes:** Staleness and linger, oxidized (metallic) taste, and bitterness.
3. **Taste defects arising from processes:** Cooked taste and caramel taste.
4. **Taste defects arising from microbial growth:** Sourness, moldy taste, cheesy taste, and fruity taste.
5. **Other cases:** Tastes resulting from external contaminants and cleaning agents.

13.2.2 Body

The body of ice cream pertains to its overall integrity and mass, while the structure relates to the microscopic makeup of the ice cream (Figure 13.2). The composition of the mixture and the degree of aeration significantly influence the body of ice cream. A relatively dense body is desirable in ice cream. Body defects in ice cream can be categorized as follows:

1. Brittle, fragile, and crumbly.
2. Gummy, chewy, adhesive, and stringy.
3. Wrinkled.
4. Heavy, doughy, pudding-like, and moist.
5. Weak and watery.

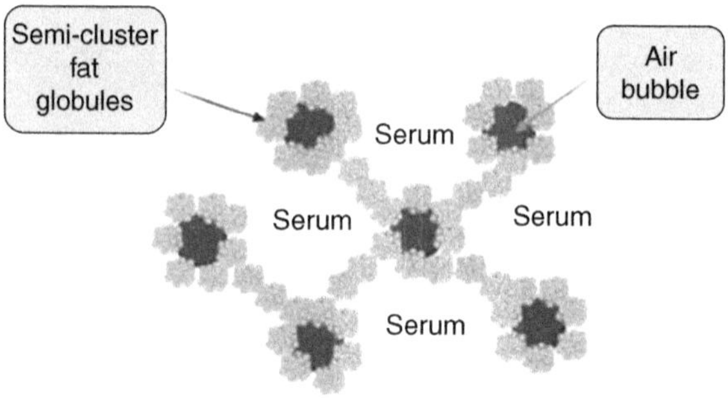

Figure 13.2 A schematic representation of the microscopic structure of ice cream (fat globules positioned within the walls of air bubbles, forming aggregates dispersed in the serum phase).

13.2.3 Texture

Texture of food products is often perceived through touch, tongue, and teeth, and it relates to the physical structure of the food. The physical structure of a food item is the result of the interaction between its chemical components and their physical properties. The examination of food texture is important from three aspects:

1. Evaluating the resistance of food products to mechanical forces, such as those encountered during mechanical handling of fruits and vegetables.
2. Determining the flow properties of food materials during processing, transportation, and storage.
3. Understanding the mechanical behavior of food materials during consumption.

Special terms are used to describe texture, and we will elaborate on them as follows:

1. **Firmness:** Pertains to rheological properties of the food material, including its fluidity and deformation.
2. **Hardness:** Used to describe resistance to deformation. Firmness is equivalent to hardness, but sometimes hardness is used specifically to denote resistance to deformation under the force of its weight.
3. **Brittleness:** The tendency of a food item to break before flowing is observed.
4. **Stickiness:** Relates to surface properties and results from the adhesion between materials and an absorbing surface. When the two surfaces are of the same material, the term cohesion is used.

5. Other terms like "dry and brittle," "oily and greasy," "smooth," "moist," "powdery," and "pulpy and fibrous" are also used to describe texture characteristics.

Measuring textural properties of food materials can be useful in process design, equipment development, and understanding consumer acceptance. Texture defects in ice cream can be categorized as follows:

1. Rough, icy, granular, and gritty.
2. Sandy and toothsome.
3. Buttery and greasy.
4. Snowy and powdery.
5. Light, fluffy, crumbly, and spongy.

13.2.4 Color

The color of ice cream should be appealing, pleasant, and reminiscent of its flavor. It must be uniformly distributed throughout the ice cream. Most consumers perceive lightly colored products as having less flavor. Therefore, color intensity plays a significant role in the perception of taste. Defects related to ice cream color can be categorized as follows:

1. Dull and hazy color.
2. Nonuniform color.
3. Excessive brightness and intense shine.
4. Faded, chalky, and color absence.
5. Unnatural color.

13.2.5 Appearance

The appearance of a product is the first criterion that influences a customer. Appearance can refer to the packaging on supermarket shelves or how the ice cream is presented inside containers on a display table. Packaging appearance matters; if the packaging does not appeal to the customer, they will not buy it. If the packaging of a product does not catch the customer's attention, the quality of the ice cream will never be evaluated. Most ice cream consumers start differentiating between ice cream qualities based on its appearance. General characteristics like the gumminess and stickiness of the texture, the roughness and iciness of the structure, the pleasing color, and the sense of goodness that represents the desired taste all impact the customer's perception. The appearance of ice cream, after it has melted, becomes less important compared to other factors. This factor usually only comes into focus when the product is undesirably grainy, and a liquid of a cheese-like color separates from it. The color of food products has a psychological influence on the acceptability of various foods by different individuals, and ice cream is no exception. Therefore, multiple quality factors related to the appearance of the product influence our perception as customers, even before we taste the product. Hence, these factors should be carefully controlled.

13.2.6 Melting

The speed of ice cream melting is one of the important quality factors for ice cream. This is particularly critical for novelty ice creams. The reason for rapid melting can be traced to a low freezing point. Slow melting is also considered defective. A quality ice cream should begin to melt at an appropriate rate and develop a flowing state, producing a soft and uniform liquid, within about 10–15 minutes at room temperature. Defects related to ice cream melting can be categorized as follows:

1. Does not melt, delayed melting, and fast melting
2. Flaky/lacks uniformity
3. Foamy-frothy/large air bubbles
4. Curdy
5. Wheying off/syneresis
6. Watery

13.2.7 Packaging

The role of packaging in sales success is undeniable. Packaging communicates the message of the packaged product to the consumer. At the same time, packaging protects the contents and enhances their shelf life. In general, packaging should be visually appealing, well-designed, and cost-effective. The color of the packaging is a significant competitive factor in the market. Drawbacks stemming from packaging can be classified as follows:

1. Slack-filled
2. Bulged
3. Misshaped
4. Improperly sealed
5. Soiled
6. Ink-smeared

References

Homayouni, A. (2013). *Functional Ice Cream: Science, Formulation and Quality Control*. Tabriz, Iran: Tabriz University of Medical Sciences.

Homayouni, A., Azizi, A., Ehsani, M.R., and Yarmand, M.S. (2008). Effect of microencapsulation and resistant starch on the probiotic survival and sensory properties of synbiotic ice cream. *Food Chemistry* 111 (1): 50–55.

Marshall, R.T., Goff, H.D., and Hartel, R.W. (2003). *Ice Cream*, 6e. New York: Kluwer Academic/Plenum Publishers.

14

Shelf-Life Evaluation of Probiotic Ice Cream

14.1 Ice Cream Shelf Life

Production of short-lived products has been common over the years. This has led the manufactured products to be sold and consumed shortly after production. After World War II, the food industry underwent significant changes in Europe, America, and Japan. These changes resulted in major alterations in the way dairy products were stored, particularly refrigeration. People's interest in new products led to the development of consumer markets and innovative marketing methods. On the other hand, food industry units focused on achieving high efficiency, reducing costs, and increasing profitability in industrial hubs. The increase in production capacity and transportation of refrigerated products, along with reduced trade restrictions in European society, improved business opportunities. As a result of this development, refrigerated dairy products, once considered perishable and sensitive, are now consumable just days after production. The rise in market demand led to various technical issues, ultimately triggering a significant transformation in food technology. Ensuring the safety of manufactured products holds significant importance. Additionally, for successful production, other food parameters must be maintained at a high level. This means that sensory, visual, and physical characteristics of the product should remain similar to fresh products at the end of their shelf life. In general, the need to preserve product freshness and safety without any artificial preservatives poses numerous challenges for food technologists. Governments have mandated the labeling of product dates as a means to ensure the quality of food items for consumers. Initially, factories used to specify the "sell-by date" on food packaging. Nowadays, according to European regulations, nonperishable food products are labeled with a "best before date," while perishable products susceptible to microbial spoilage, such as dairy desserts, are labeled with a "use-by date" (expiration date).

Probiotic Ice Cream: Science and Technology, First Edition. Aziz Homayouni-Rad.

Furthermore, these regulations compel manufacturers to substantiate the claimed expiration date on their products. Therefore, manufacturers, in addition to extending the shelf life of their products, are obliged to develop methods for determining product longevity (Homayouni 2013).

14.2 Factors Affecting Ice Cream Shelf Life

From an industrial perspective, the shelf life of a food product can be defined as the number of days that a product remains consumable and maintains its quality and safety after production, meeting consumer expectations. In other words, the product must retain its microbiological health and organoleptic qualities. To determine the shelf life of a product, the characteristics of raw materials, processing methods, and storage conditions must be taken into account. The shelf life of refrigerated dairy products is influenced by the following factors:

1. **Raw materials:** The quality and properties of the raw materials used in production play a significant role in determining shelf life.
2. **Product formulation:** The specific formulation of the product, including the types and amounts of ingredients used, affects how well the product can maintain its quality over time.
3. **Processing conditions:** The processing methods employed during production, such as pasteurization or homogenization, impact the shelf life of the product.
4. **Adherence to good manufacturing practices:** Following proper manufacturing conditions and hygiene practices contributes to extending shelf life.
5. **Packaging:** The type and quality of packaging used can significantly affect the product's exposure to external factors like air, light, and moisture.
6. **Storage and distribution conditions:** The conditions under which the product is stored and transported can influence its shelf life. Factors like temperature control during storage and transportation are crucial.
7. **Consumption conditions:** How the product is handled and consumed by the end consumer also plays a role in its shelf life. For example, proper refrigeration and adherence to usage instructions can impact how long the product remains safe and of high quality.

In the food industry, determining and ensuring the appropriate shelf life involves carefully considering all of these factors and conducting tests and studies to validate the product's safety and quality over time. Measurement, recording, and control of the above factors hold primary importance in assessing shelf life. The point at which a product becomes unacceptable in terms of organoleptic or microbiological aspects is considered the endpoint of shelf life.

14.2.1 Raw Materials

The raw materials used in the production of ice cream and frozen desserts include milk, cream, milk solids, starter cultures, sweeteners, flavorings, emulsifiers, stabilizers, colors, and bakery products like cakes and biscuits. Each of these materials can carry microbes and chemical substances, thereby affecting the quality of the final product. Consequently, raw materials should be sourced from reliable and approved sources to ensure that the product maintains consistent quality and shelf life. Any alteration in raw materials or sourcing centers can impact the product's shelf life (Marshall et al. 2003).

14.2.1.1 Milk

Milk is a common base for all dairy products. The composition of milk, including protein, fat, lactose, and microbial flora, is variable. Different stages of milking, geographical shifts, and seasonal changes all have a considerable impact on milk composition. Controlling the type and quantity of microbes and the protein content of milk is of utmost importance for the stability of the final product's texture and shelf life. Microbes can enter milk through cows, workers, dairy equipment, transportation and storage equipment, as well as processing equipment. To minimize the microbial load in milk, its temperature must be immediately reduced to below 5°C right after milking. Typically, milk is stored at this temperature prior to processing in the factory. Some large factories have collection centers where milk is sent to the factory once every day or even twice a week. These facilities encourage dairy farmers to implement hygienic practices in milking and storage. Nonetheless, microbial growth and enzymatic activity in these milks are still significant. Modern processing methods and existing national standards have led to the use of high-quality milk in dairy product formulations. This milk has good taste, low microbial load, and is free from any impurities. Upon arrival at the factory, high-quality milk is immediately subjected to heat treatment and cooled to around 5°C to prevent further deterioration due to storage. Therefore, milk used in dairy product formulations should have a low microbial load, be free from undesirable flavors, and have a minimal enzymatic breakdown. Proper management of stored milk circulation and temperature control helps maintain the quality of raw milk.

14.2.1.2 Cream

The quality of cream depends on the quality of the milk used for cream separation and the method of cream handling before and after pasteurization. Cream is sensitive to enzymatic hydrolysis due to its high-fat content. Lipase enzyme hydrolyzes triglycerides into fatty acids, mono- and diglycerides, and glycerol. This process leads to the development of a rancid (sour) taste in the final product. Lipase is largely inactivated during pasteurization. However, as many microorganisms produce lipase, this can be problematic for cream that is handled unhygienically after transportation. If the milk brought to the factory has been stored for an extended period before cream separation, it is immediately pasteurized upon reception. Microbial quality is measured and recorded through total viable count (TVC) and total coliform count.

14.2.1.3 Condensed Milk

Two common methods are typically used to produce condensed milk from milk solids:

(1) **Water evaporation:** Water is removed through evaporation.
(2) **Membrane filtration:** Water is removed through membrane filtration.

In both cases, the quality of condensed milk depends on the quality of the milk used and the handling techniques before and during the process. The microbial load of the milk, especially heat-resistant bacteria (thermoduric) and spores, should be low. Additionally, the milk should have sufficient chemical stability for heat treatment. After concentration, temperature control and handling methods are crucial for the microbial quality of condensed milk. The crystallization of lactose, depending on the cooling rate and concentration factor, can occur and impact the flavor and texture of the final product. Microbiological quality is assessed through the counting of spore-forming bacteria and coliforms, while chemical quality is monitored through measurements of fat, lactose, protein, solids, and pH.

14.2.1.4 Starter Culture

Controlling the activity and viability of starter microorganisms is essential for achieving the quality and shelf life of fermented products. The preparation, transportation, and transfer of starter cultures require adherence to sanitary standards and awareness of production techniques. Contamination from molds, yeasts, bacteria, and bacteriophages must be prevented. Starter inoculum, when used, should contain a high number of live and active bacteria in the appropriate ratio to achieve the desired pH within the specified time. The quality of the provided starter culture can be maintained by storing it at temperatures below 5°C for a maximum of 48 hours. The quality of the starter culture can be controlled through tests for mold, yeast, cellular balance (ratio), and its activity. Direct inoculation from frozen cells is used, and these cells must be stored at very low temperatures and utilized according to the manufacturer's instructions. Maintaining the vitality and quality of the starter culture is crucial for consistent and desirable fermentation processes in dairy product production.

14.2.1.5 Fruits

Fruits are capable of being preserved for a limited period of time after harvest. The duration of preservation depends on the type of fruit, variety, geographical location, harvesting method, and storage conditions. Fruit spoilage occurs due to microbial activity, especially when the fruit is damaged, and chemical reactions catalyzed by enzymes take place. To maintain the quality of fruits, it is necessary to combat factors that lead to spoilage. This can be achieved through methods such as thermal sterilization (canning) or deep freezing. These processes help in preserving the quality and extending the shelf life of fruits.

14.2.1.6 Other Raw Materials

The composition of food, the sources of these materials, the reliability of suppliers, identifying critical control points, and hygiene standards all play a significant role in the shelf life of the final product. Proper selection and management of all raw materials used in food production contribute to the overall quality and longevity of the end product.

14.3 Shelf Life of Frozen Foods

14.3.1 Effect of Microorganisms

Microbial growth is significantly slowed down at temperatures ranging from −8 to 0°C. In this temperature range, microbial activity experiences drastic physical and chemical changes. Consequently, microbial spoilage is halted within the temperature range of −12 to −9°C. However, the enzymes present in these microorganisms remain active and still contribute to some extent to food spoilage. Processed foods that have been blanched or cooked and then properly frozen tend to have a longer shelf life compared to raw frozen foods. Pathogenic bacteria like *Salmonella*, *Clostridium perfringens* spores, and *Escherichia coli* tend to undergo logarithmic reductions during long-term cold storage in a freezer. This means their numbers decrease exponentially over time. Proper freezing and storage temperatures are crucial in preventing the growth of harmful microorganisms and maintaining the quality and safety of frozen foods.

14.3.2 Movement of Ice Crystals in Food Systems

When the temperature drops below −18°C, ice crystals become a part of the food's structure. These ice crystals are unstable due to changes in water vapor pressure caused by temperature gradients. Therefore, to maintain the stability of ice crystals (in terms of shape and size), the distribution of frozen food must occur at a constant temperature. Temperature fluctuations within the range of 2–3°C during storage of the product at −18°C or lower, even over a long period of time, do not cause significant damage to the food. However, repeated temperature changes, especially in the range of −5 to −1°C, where severe ice crystal formation occurs, can lead to the growth, aggregation, and clustering of ice crystals. These ice crystals can migrate to the surface of the food product and even to the surface of the packaging material if suitable space is present. This phenomenon often occurs during the distribution of frozen food by street vendors and during transportation of the food to homes. In such cases, if the packaging material is permeable to moisture, water gradually exits the food material or moves as vapor out of the packaging. As a result, the food material loses moisture under freezing conditions, leading to the drying out of the product. The loss of moisture causes animal tissues to become firmer, and increased contact between the product and the oxygen present in the packaging occurs. Oxygen triggers unfavorable changes in frozen foods, such as oxidation of unsaturated lipids, color degradation, and the development of off-flavors. These changes are attributed to the oxygen present within the packaging.

14.3.3 Physicochemical Reactions

Various physicochemical reactions occur in frozen products that can lead to changes in flavor, degradation of vitamins, alteration of protein nature, hydrolysis in dairy products, and oxidation-related deterioration. Additionally, the crystallization of sugars, such as sucrose (especially at temperatures around −23°C where it occurs at a maximum rate), and lactose crystallization (which results in a gritty texture in ice cream) are among the physicochemical reactions in frozen products. Nucleation, crystal growth, changes in the rate of thawing and thawing release, and other quality defects play a significant role in determining the shelf life of frozen products. Therefore, formulation and food processing should be designed in a way that minimizes these mentioned changes.

14.3.4 Time-Temperature Tolerance (TTT)

Studying the time-temperature tolerance (TTT) of frozen food products under different temperature-time conditions reveals that the quality and shelf life of the food are dependent on the storage temperature. The quality stability of frozen foods during storage follows the Arrhenius equation.

14.3.5 PPP Factors (Product Quality, Processing, and Packaging)

The inherent quality of food components (freshness and freezability), processing (enzyme inactivation, cooking, chopping, and adding antioxidants), and packaging (oxygen and moisture permeability), as well as the degree of vacuum (composition of gases within it), determine the final product quality. These factors complicate the determination of shelf life using the TTT approach.

14.3.6 Glass Transition State

As previously mentioned, the concept of TTT is used to determine the shelf life of frozen food products. By identifying the PPP factors, these factors are also incorporated into the determination of shelf life, and the TTT and PPP theories have been reviewed and complimented. With decreasing temperature, more of the water present in the food enters a crystalline state and the remaining solution becomes more concentrated. The viscosity of the solution increases with its increasing concentration. Eventually, a point is reached where the food reaches the glass transition temperature (Tg). At this temperature, the materials present between ice crystals (the concentrated solution) transition into a glassy state. In this state, an amorphous, highly stable solid with a very high viscosity (above 10^{13} pascal-seconds) and an irregular liquid-like structure is formed. The transition from a viscoelastic fluid state to a glassy state results in a significant reduction in the movement of ice crystals (and other components). As a result, the speed of all reactions decreases, and the decline in quality comes to a halt. The Tg of ice cream varies depending on its formulation, ranging from approximately −23 to −43°C. The moisture content has a minor effect on the Tg. The presence of small molecular solutes like sugars decreases the Tg. While high molecular weight components like starch have a small effect on Tg. The rate of quality decline at temperatures above Tg depends on the difference between the cold storage temperature and Tg. Understanding the Tgs of frozen food materials and the factors affecting them enables researchers to optimize food formulations and production processes to have a higher Tg (warmer temperature). Therefore, selecting a cold storage temperature for frozen food products based on Tg preserves product quality and saves energy consumption. Lowering the storage temperature below Tg increases energy costs. If the temperature exceeds the Tg threshold, quality deterioration occurs.

14.3.7 Knowledge About the Product

A prerequisite for planning the determination of the shelf life of a frozen product is selecting a temperature-sensitive characteristic of that product. This characteristic could be factors such as flavor deterioration, color change, rancidity, and so on. Evaluation of each of these characteristics is carried out by trained evaluation groups. Sometimes, it is also possible to estimate the shelf life of a product from similar products of other companies.

14.3.8 Targeted Tests

In certain frozen products, specific tests are employed to control quality. These tests rarely reflect customer preferences and are used less frequently to determine product shelf life. Among these tests, we can mention assays for assessing nutritional value degradation, such as vitamin C degradation, or tests for determining peroxide value in products containing unsaturated lipids. The results of these tests can somewhat predict the outcomes of sensory evaluations.

14.3.9 Accelerated Tests

The deterioration of quality in frozen foods is a gradual process, and quality changes occur at a slower, irreversible pace. The decline in quality of frozen foods happens more rapidly at higher temperatures compared to lower temperatures. In other words, Q_{10} these reactions are always positive, Q_{10} indicating that the quality deterioration ratio at two different temperatures, typically situated within the range of frozen food storage temperatures and differing by approximately 10°C, is consistently positive. However, Q_{10} not all frozen foods adhere to this pattern. Q_{10} A value of one is assigned to products that are temperature-indifferent and exhibit neutral stability (e.g. Salami). The quality of these products, such as processed cheese, fermented, and dried products, is not dependent on temperature. Such a product has a longer shelf life in freezing temperatures compared to refrigeration and ambient temperatures. Q_{10} Negative values are rarely observed in foods. For instance, processed pork products that are vacuum-sealed, like

Bacon, have a longer shelf life at −5°C compared to −25°C. In this case, with further temperature reduction and increased frozen water content, catalysts such as sodium chloride, nitrates, and nitrites concentrate in the nonfrozen phase, leading to oxidative rancidity. Accelerated tests involve keeping a control sample at −40°C or below and subjecting other samples to treatments at three or four different temperatures ranging from −30 to −10°C. In most cases, the control sample is kept at −30°C, and the remaining samples are placed at higher temperatures. This is because fewer changes occur in the control sample at −30°C. Since various fruits are used in ice cream formulations, factors such as vitamin C degradation, flavor reduction, and color loss can be utilized as indicators of quality deterioration.

14.3.10 Cold Chain

When determining the shelf life of a frozen product, it is important to consider that a food product is not consistently held at a single temperature (e.g. −25°C) from freezing until consumption. Ice cream, for instance, goes through several stages after freezing and before consumption. It spends some time in a cold storage room below −25°C, then is transported in refrigerated trucks, kept in a refrigerator after distribution, and finally displayed for sale. After purchase, the customer takes the ice cream home at ambient temperature and may store it in their household freezer for a period. All these transfers involve temperature changes and could entail relatively significant temperature fluctuations during these stages, ultimately impacting the quality of the final product. Sometimes, the quality of the ice cream received by the consumer can vary drastically from the ice cream produced in the factory in terms of quality. Figure 14.1 illustrates a temperature profile of a sample cold chain process in Europe.

By placing thermometers inside the compartments where ice cream is stored during various transportation stages, you can control the product's temperature from production to transportation and distribution to consumption. These thermometers can record the ambient temperature around them every 15 minutes. Additionally, nowadays, temperature-time indicators are used in different distribution stages. Another significant tool for enhancing the shelf life of frozen food products is controlling storage time. Through proper formulation, processing, packaging, and storage at appropriate temperatures, you can extend the product's shelf life. Adhering to the "first-in-first-out" (FIFO) principle, the product that entered the storage first should also leave the storage before others, reaching the consumer's hands. This ensures that products are consumed before their expiration dates.

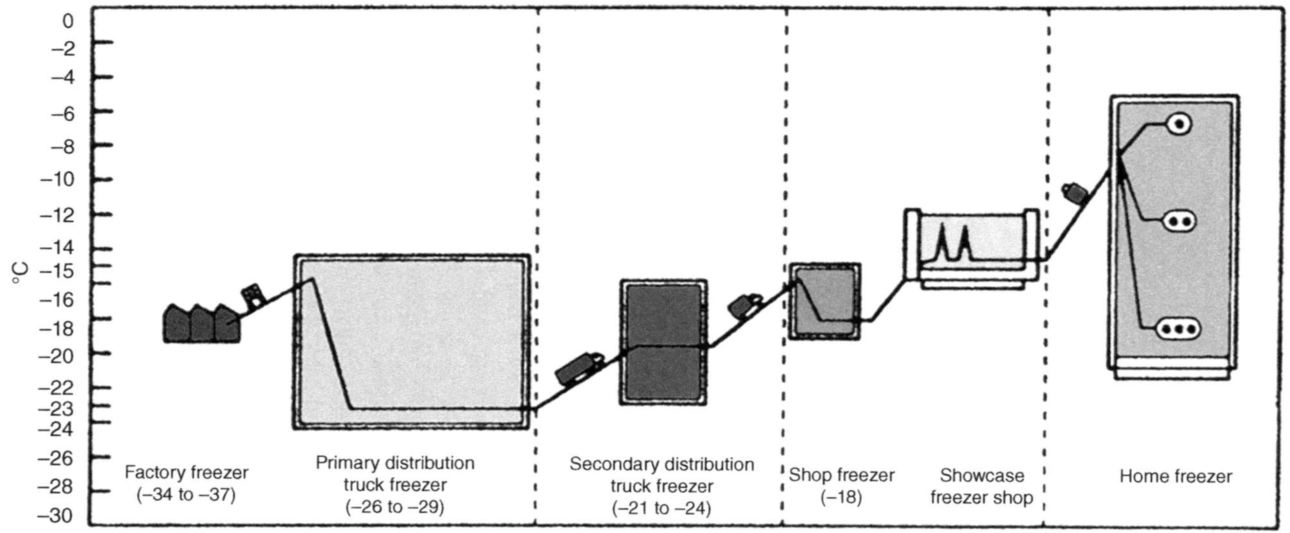

Figure 14.1 Temperature profile of a sample cold chain process.

14.4 Determining Shelf Life in Practice

In this section, we will explore the process of determining the shelf life of frozen products through an example. The methodology used in this example can also be applied to other frozen dairy products. Frozen dairy products fall into the category of products with extended shelf life.

14.4.1 Determining Shelf Life with Storage Tests

To determine the shelf life of a product, samples are held under specific conditions. The storage conditions for achieving the desired shelf life include:

1. The control sample is fully frozen at −30°C.
2. Under average storage conditions, one of the treatments is placed at −18°C.
3. Under average storage conditions and for accelerated shelf life determination, treatments are kept at −12, −6, and −2°C (refrigerator). The duration of product storage under these conditions is 18 months, while a shelf life of 12 months is desired and sufficient for consumers.

The experimental design, sample collection, and testing procedures should follow a specific plan. In this example, sampling is performed every two months. This way, control and average storage condition treatments are sampled at 0, 2, 4, 6, 8, 10, 12, 14, 16, and 18 months, and necessary tests are conducted on these samples. For treatments held under the worst possible conditions, samples are collected after three days, one week, and one month. The tests used to determine the impact of storage time on product quality include:

1. Moisture loss assessment by weighing the product after removing it from its packaging.
2. Sensory evaluation by a panel of five individuals familiar with the product's characteristics. Evaluations are done using a seven-point Hedonic scale where one is "completely unacceptable," four is "average," and seven is "completely acceptable" (control). They assess the product's appearance, texture, overall acceptability, and meltability. During the evaluation, both the average and the worst sample compared to the control are identified, and a seven-point Hedonic scale is then used for precise evaluation. Sensory evaluation tests should be designed to focus on customer-friendly and market-friendly attributes.

The minimum required number of samples for evaluation is as follows:

1. One package of each control and average storage condition treatment is required for sensory evaluation. Thus, over the 18-month storage period, a total of 19 product packages will be needed.
2. Three packages of each accelerated storage condition treatment (accelerated conditions) are required for sensory evaluation. Thus, a total of nine product packages will be needed.
3. In total, 28 packages are needed for evaluation. However, for extra caution, it is better to take more samples to ensure safety margins (double the total samples). The control and average storage condition samples are initially weighed, coded, and then placed in boxes for storage. It is advisable to analyze the data immediately after collection and plot the relevant graph. Additionally, alongside these tests, an extra test should be conducted on one of the normally stored packages in storage.

14.4.2 Ice Cream Shelf Life

One of the major drawbacks of ice cream is the development of a coarse and icy texture. The formation of ice crystals in the ice cream is the primary factor limiting its shelf life, causing significant damage to its quality. Nowadays, the causes of ice crystallization and the influencing factors have been identified. "Ice cream shelf life" does not have a fixed time range and is often dependent on storage conditions. The shelf life of ice cream can vary from two weeks to a year. Among the methods to prevent ice crystallization in ice cream, suitable formulation, rapid freezing, and firming, as well as avoiding temperature fluctuations during storage and distribution, are noteworthy. The more numerous and smaller and uniform the ice crystals are, the less they are perceptible in the mouth. Thermal shock and significant temperature fluctuations can lead to the disappearance of fine and uniform ice crystals, resulting in a coarse and icy texture in ice cream. Increasing the awareness of both sellers and consumers of ice cream about the causes of ice crystallization and how to prevent it can aid in maintaining a smooth texture of the product.

14.4.2.1 Effect of Temperature Fluctuations and Ice Crystal Recrystallization on Shelf Life

Ice crystals in ice cream are usually unstable, and changes in their number, size, and shape occur during the storage period in the freezer. This phenomenon is known as recrystallization. This phenomenon is often considered the most significant factor contributing to quality degradation in frozen food products. While ice crystal recrystallization naturally occurs at a constant temperature, it becomes more pronounced when temperature fluctuations are present. If the temperature of the ice cream increases during its storage in the freezer, some of the ice crystals, especially the finer ones, melt, increasing the amount of unfrozen water in the serum phase. Conversely, as the temperature decreases, the water freezes, but this time new ice nuclei are not formed, and the water freezes onto the surface of larger ice crystals. As a result of recrystallization, the number of ice crystals decreases, and their average size increases. Temperature fluctuations during the storage period in the freezer are inevitable. This is due to the fact that refrigeration systems operate periodically and intermittently, and snow buildup occasionally needs to be removed from the surface of these systems, which often involves turning off the systems. However, incorrect handling of the product during transportation is considered the main cause of recrystallization. Turning off the refrigeration units of distribution trucks, supermarket refrigerators, vending equipment, and even the consumer's shopping basket until the product reaches home are among the most critical points of temperature fluctuations. Plotting the temperature changes during distribution, supply, and consumption clearly highlights this point. Therefore, maintaining a consistently low temperature can minimize ice crystal recrystallization.

14.4.2.2 Role of Stabilizers in Shelf Life

Stabilizers such as locust bean gum, guar gum, carboxymethyl cellulose, sodium alginate, carrageenan, and xanthan gum are commonly used in ice cream formulation. These substances are often available in ready-to-use blends on the market, usually in combination with emulsifiers. The purpose of adding stabilizers to ice cream is to create a smooth and creamy texture, prevent or delay the growth of ice crystals and lactose during the product's storage in the freezer, and ensure uniformity, and resistance to melting. Additionally, stabilizers can prevent the separation of the serum phase from the ice cream mixture and create a stable foam that allows the product to be easily scooped from the freezer. Stabilizers also prevent moisture migration from the product into the packaging or the air. The mechanism of action of these polysaccharides is related to the formation of a gel-like structure that traps and binds free water. The control of ice crystal growth by stabilizers is likely associated with the reduction in the mobility of water trapped within the three-dimensional network structure of the serum phase. Proper ice cream formulation with stabilizers is one of the main ways to prevent the growth of inevitable ice crystals during heat shock. The importance of stabilizers in ice cream lies in their ability to counteract the increase in sugar and lactose content, which would otherwise promote the recrystallization of these components. On the other hand, a small amount of solid ingredients in the ice cream mixture leads to an increase in free water, resulting in more ice crystals present at any given temperature.

14.4.2.3 Role of Communication in Ice Cream Shelf Life

Raising awareness among distributors, retailers, and ice cream consumers about heat shock and textural changes in the product, as well as how to prevent them, is of great importance. Although control of the product, after it leaves the factory, is beyond the control of the manufacturer, it should not be forgotten that consumers purchase the product with the brand name of the manufacturer. The quality of the product, regardless of when and where a defect occurs, affects the credibility of the manufacturer in the eyes of the consumer. Consumers should be informed that ice cream is unlike other frozen products and requires specific conditions for transportation and storage. Communication efforts play a crucial role in educating consumers and all stakeholders about the unique nature of ice cream and its sensitivity to temperature fluctuations. Distributors and retailers should be well-informed about the proper handling and storage of ice cream to ensure that the product maintains its quality throughout the distribution chain. This can include guidelines on maintaining consistent freezer temperatures, avoiding temperature fluctuations, and handling the product with care to prevent excessive exposure to warm air. Furthermore, consumers should be educated about the best practices for storing ice cream at home, such as keeping it in the coldest part of the freezer, avoiding frequent opening and closing of the freezer door, and consuming the product before its expiration date. This knowledge empowers consumers to make informed decisions that contribute to preserving the quality and shelf life of the ice cream they purchase. In summary, effective communication not only helps maintain the reputation of ice cream manufacturers but also empowers distributors, retailers, and consumers to play a proactive role in preserving the quality and shelf life of ice cream from production to consumption.

14.4.2.4 Methods to Increase Ice Cream Shelf Life

(a) **Effective formulation:** Creating a well-formulated ice cream recipe that takes into account stabilizers and the impact of sugars on freezing point depression is essential. Proper formulation can enhance the texture, prevent ice crystal formation, and extend shelf life.

(b) **Quick freezing:** Rapid freezing of ice cream helps in producing small ice crystals and maintaining a smooth texture. Proper maintenance and care of freezers are crucial. Continuous-use freezers with high heat exchange rates, preventing refrigerant line blockages by oil, regular maintenance of freezer blades, reducing the distance between packaging and freezer, and prechilling the ice cream mix before freezing are effective strategies.

(c) **Rapid hardening:** Ensuring that the ice cream hardens quickly after freezing can improve its shelf life. Techniques like heat exchangers with agitation and forcing cold compressed air into the hardening process can help. Increasing the temperature difference between the product and the cooling medium, avoiding stacking cartons in the freezer to allow proper air circulation, and shrink-wrapping the product containers (using polymer coatings like nylon) can also aid in rapid hardening.

(d) **Temperature control:** Preventing temperature fluctuations during storage and distribution is crucial. Maintaining lower temperatures as much as possible and ensuring temperature stability until the product reaches the consumer is important. Avoiding improper handling of products after packaging, such as stacking them in the production area before transfer to the freezer, is essential.

(e) **Education:** Educating retailers and consumers about ice cream shelf life is vital. Retailers should be informed about proper storage and handling practices to maintain the quality of the product. Consumers should be educated about the importance of proper home storage, consuming the product before its expiration date, and avoiding temperature abuse.

Incorporating these methods into the ice cream production and distribution process can help extend the shelf life of the product while maintaining its desired quality and texture.

References

Homayouni, A. (2013). *Functional Ice Cream: Science, Formulation and Quality Control*. Tabriz, Iran: Tabriz University of Medical Sciences.

Marshall, R.T., Goff, H.D., and Hartel, R.W. (2003). *Ice Cream*, 6e. New York: Kluwer Academic/Plenum Publishers.

Index

Note: *Italicized* and **bold** page numbers refer to figures and tables, respectively.

Probiotic Ice Cream: Science and Technology, First Edition. Aziz Homayouni-Rad.

g

n

o

p

Printed in the USA/Agawam, MA
September 16, 2026

910661.179